HEALTH AND WELL-BEING FOR INTERIOR ARCHITECTURE

With fifteen essays by scholars and professionals, from fields such as policy and law, *Health and Well-being for Interior Architecture* asks readers to consider climate, geography, and culture alongside human biology, psychology, and sociology. Since designers play such a pivotal role in human interaction with interior and architectural design, this book sheds light on the importance of a designer's attention to health and well-being while also acknowledging the ever changing built environment. Through various viewpoints, and over 30 images, this book guides designers through ways to create and develop interior designs in order to improve occupants' health and well-being.

Dak Kopec is an Associate Professor in the School of Architecture at the University of Nevada, Las Vegas. He has a Ph.D. in Environmental Psychology and graduate degrees in Community Psychology and Architecture. He is also certified by the National Commission of Health Education Credentialing at the Masters level. His specialties include custom housing for people with specific health conditions, and designs for community-based organizations, social service agencies, and educational facilities for underserved populations.

'*Health and Well-being for Interior Architecture* is a much-needed book for the healthcare design industry. The strength of this book is its focus on health and wellness across the lifespan and how the environment affects the human experience and sense of well-being in various settings – schools, residential environments, birthing environments, and healthcare settings. The chapters are written by well-known experts in their fields lending tremendous credibility to this important book.'

—**Jaynelle F. Stichler**, DNS, RN, NEA-BC, EDAC, FACHE, FAAN, Co-Editor of *HERD Journal,* Professor Emerita, School of Nursing, San Diego State University, San Diego, California, USA

'Dak Kopec brings together an international set of respected experts whose research offers crucial ways of thinking about design for human habitation through all stages of life: from places of birth and schools to spaces where we can work safely, develop spiritually, and age gracefully. Readers will recognize the multifarious influence environments have on human health and how concerns for social justice—including strategies for making adaptable and contaminant-free places—are integral to ensuring a better future across our fragile globe. This volume enlarges our knowledge about the designer's main task: creating healthy and sustainable places that enrich and reinforce well-being for all.'

—**William T. Willoughby**, AIA, Associate Professor and Associate Dean, College of Architecture and Environmental Design, Kent State University, Kent, Ohio, USA

'This timely book provides an integrated cross-disciplinary view of design issues fundamental to the collaborative conceptualization of effective design strategies to support healthy cognitive and physical functioning. It is an informative reference for students as well as professional practitioners in the healthcare design industry and related disciplines. It will be an excellent user-friendly textbook for beginning and intermediate students.'

—**Attila Lawrence**, Professor and Program Coordinator, Master of Healthcare Interior Design Program, Bachelor of Science Interior Architecture and Design Program, School of Architecture, University of Nevada, Las Vegas

'This publication brings together important perspectives on wellbeing, spanning cultures and integrating diverse schools of thought. It uniquely addresses the complexity of health as it is related to the build environment including traditional and contemporary approaches to healing, lifestyle and empathy, legal issues and environmental pathogens. The contributors highlight both the complexity of human wellbeing alongside the inseparable role of the made environment. This collection offers important perspectives regardless of experience level or profession.'

—**Jennifer Webb**, Ph.D., NCIDQ, LEED AP., Associate Professor, Department of Interior Design, Fay Jones School of Architecture and Design, University of Arkansas

'*Health and Well-being for Interior Architecture* is an important resource for practitioners of many professions: designers, clinicians, and social scientists. This book is packed with interesting and diverse ideas that are timely and relevant for greater discussion and application. Throughout the book there are many crucial issues that have been thoroughly addressed in this very readable text. Timely, important, and accessible makes this text a must have for practicing professionals.'

—**Sally Augustin**, PhD., Principal, Design With Science, Editor, Research Design Connections

HEALTH AND WELL-BEING FOR INTERIOR ARCHITECTURE

Edited by Dak Kopec

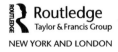

Routledge
Taylor & Francis Group

NEW YORK AND LONDON

First published 2017
by Routledge
711 Third Avenue, New York, NY 10017

and by Routledge
2 Park Square, Milton Park, Abingdon, Oxon OX14 4RN

Routledge is an imprint of the Taylor & Francis Group, an informa business

© 2017 Taylor & Francis

The right of the editor Dak Kopec to be identified as the author of the editorial material, and of the authors for their individual chapters, has been asserted in accordance with sections 77 and 78 of the Copyright, Designs and Patents Act 1988.

Library of Congress Cataloguing-in-Publication Data
A catalog record for this book has been requested

ISBN: 978-1-138-20661-8 (hbk)
ISBN: 978-1-138-20662-5 (pbk)
ISBN: 978-1-315-46441-1 (ebk)

Typeset in Bembo
by Apex CoVantage, LLC

This book is dedicated to all of the amazing authors who contributed to this publication. Their expertise, professionalism, and flexibility made this one of the best projects I have ever worked on! THANK YOU!

CONTENTS

CONTRIBUTORS

Sherry Ahrentzen, Ph.D., is Shimberg Professor of Housing Studies at the University of Florida. Her research focuses on housing and community design that fosters the physical, social and economic health of households. Her recent work examined the impacts of green building practices on resident health and indoor environmental quality in housing of low-income older adults. In 2013, she received the James Haecker Award for Distinguished Leadership in Architectural Research.

Sharon Cook is a Senior Lecturer in Ergonomics with a specialist interest in Inclusive Design at Loughborough University in the UK. She has pioneered the development of wearable simulations of aging and disability as a form of empathic modeling thereby raising awareness of inclusivity within industry and promoting improved product and service design. She was awarded the UK's Chartered Institute of Ergonomics and Human Factors Ergonomics Design Award in recognition of excellence in her application of ergonomics to design.

Shauna Corry Hernandez earned a Master of Arts in Interior Design (1990) and an Interdisciplinary Ph.D. focusing on Environment and Behavior (2002) from Washington State University. She is currently an associate professor and Interim Dean of the College of Art and Architecture at the University of Idaho where she has served as Interior Design Program Coordinator and Program Head. Currently, she serves as a Director on the Interior Design Educators Council Foundation Board and is a past IDEC Pacific West Regional Chair. Universal design and social justice are her research interests, and she has presented at national and international conferences.

Lynne M. Dearborn, Ph.D., is Associate Professor at the University of Illinois' Urbana campus and a member of the School of Architecture's health and well-being program. She advises Ph.D. students in architecture and landscape architecture and teaches survey of design and health research. Her work explores questions of social justice and equity among minority peoples, engaging physical, social, economic, and political aspects of the environment to address human health and well-being.

Nicole DeNamur, J.D., WELL AP™, LEED® Green Associate™, is a Seattle-based attorney with Pacifica Law Group whose practice focuses on insurance coverage and construction litigation. She is also an Affiliate Instructor at the University of Washington's Runstad Center for Real Estate Studies, where she developed the Multidisciplinary course entitled *Risk and Reward in Sustainable Development*. Nicole regularly presents on her proactive approach to risk management and the legal issues associated with sustainable building design, construction and operations.

Moira Gannon Denson, ASID, IDEC, LEED AP, is an Assistant Professor of Interior Design and graduate student advisor at Marymount University and an NCIDQ-certified Interior Designer. Her professional experience is in project delivery and interdisciplinary coordination of health care, workplace, hospitality, and residential building types at firms such as Gordon and Greenberg Architects, Design Collective Inc., and most recently Perkins + Will.

Carole Després is a professor of architecture at Laval University in Québec City, Canada, and holds a Ph.D. in Environment-Behavior Studies. She is the director and co-founder of the GIRBa whose mission is to understand and act on aging suburbs in relationship to demographic change, infrastructure wear, and the need for sustainable redevelopment. Her current interests include healthy lifestyles and well-being along the life course, with ongoing action research on postwar school buildings, as well as late life housing and care.

Eugenia Victoria Ellis, AIA, is an Associate Professor at Drexel University. She holds degrees from the University of Illinois at Chicago (B.Arch.), the University of Pennsylvania (M.S.), and Virginia Tech (Ph.D.). Director of the dLUX light lab, she specializes in the visual and non-visual effects of light on design to promote occupant health and low-energy use. Her research includes daylighting, spatial visualization, visual perception, and altered states of perception, such as blindness and dementia.

James Erickson is a designer, architect, and environmentalist. He enjoys exploring new ways for our built environment to relate harmoniously with the natural landscape, integrating our communities within the planet's natural systems, and creating healthy environments for sustainable living. Dr. Erickson has a Master of Architecture from Montana State University, MSc in energy studies from the Architecture Association School of Architecture, and a Ph.D. in environmental design and planning from Arizona State University.

Maralyn J. Foureur is a Professor of Midwifery at the Faculty of Health, University of Technology Sydney. She has a particular interest in the neurophysiology of childbirth and the impact of intrapartum maternal stress on the epigenome of the baby. For the past decade her research has focused on the way the birth environment impacts on mothers, their supporters, and their care providers to either increase stress leading to pathology or to optimize wellness leading to physiological childbirth.

J. Davis Harte is a design-environment-behavior researcher and Graduate faculty member at the Boston Architectural College. She conducts translational research into uniquely authentic child-, family-, and community-centric spaces. Her Design & Human Environment MSc investigated preschool children's attentional behaviors based on the presence of houseplants. Davis conducted a video-ethnographic exploration of the experiences of childbirth supporters, as influenced by birth unit design for her Ph.D. in Health from the University of Technology Sydney.

Amanda Hatherly is the Director of the EnergySmart Academy at Santa Fe Community College where she teaches classes on energy efficiency and environmental health. She has taught a graduate class in Environmental Health for Boston Architecture College and has been a member of the National Center for Healthy Housing Curriculum Committee, developing curricula for healthy housing initiatives. Amanda speaks at conferences regularly, including the MIT Women in Clean Energy Conference and National Home Performance conference.

Sue Hignett is Professor of Healthcare Ergonomics & Patient Safety at Loughborough University (UK). She has experienced the health care industry as a clinician, ergonomist, researcher, and patient. Her research is centered on human factors and ergonomics for safer systems, emergency and CBRNe response, and staff well-being. Prof. Hignett is an Editor for 'Ergonomics'; Chair of the Education & Training panel at the Chartered Institute of Ergonomics and Human Factors; and past Chair of International Ergonomics Association Technical Committee on Healthcare Ergonomics.

Migette L. Kaup is a professor in the Department of Apparel, Textiles, and Interior Design and the Center on Aging in the College of Human Ecology at Kansas State University. She holds degrees in Interior Design and Architecture with emphasis in environment and behavior place studies, gerontology, and long-term care policy structures. Her research focuses on gerontological design, organizational development, evidence-based design strategies, and design research, specifically related to long-term care and person-centered care practices.

Robin Toft Klar, DNSc, RN, is a clinical assistant professor at NYU Meyers College of Nursing. Her interest in environmental health has evolved and currently focuses on the built environment. Her post-doc research in Global Health examined ways people in Papua New Guinea could prevent further disability from the mosquito transmitted, neglected tropical disease lymphatic filariasis. Her current focus on global workforce highlights infectious disease transmission and prevention using built environment design.

Andrée-Anne Larivière-Lajoie, M. Arch, is a graduate student in Architectural Sciences at Laval University's School of Architecture in Quebec, Canada. She is currently developing of a self-assessment tool to evaluate the quality of spaces dedicated to eating in primary schools of Quebec. She is actively involved in the Groupe Interdisciplinaire sur les Banlieues (GIRBa), and participated in several national and international conference related to her research.

Roderick J. Lawrence has a Master Degree from the University of Cambridge (England) and a Doctorate of Science from the EPFL, Lausanne, Switzerland. He is Emeritus Professor at the University of Geneva, Switzerland, Honorary Adjunct Professor at the School of Architecture and the Built Environment at the University of Adelaide, Australia, and Adjunct Professor at the Universiti Kebangsaan Malaysia. His research fields include projects funded by the European Commission and the World Health Organization on housing and urban health from a human ecology perspective; and transdisciplinary research for housing and urban planning.

Marianne Legault is a student in the Master of Architecture program at Laval University's School of Architecture in Quebec, Canada. She was involved as a research assistant in a study on the modernization of primary schools in Quebec with regard to the integration of afterschool care, under the supervision of Carole Després. She is a member of the Groupe Interdisciplinaire sur les Banlieues (GIRBa) and has contributed to several presentations on this subject.

Sandrine Tremblay-Lemieux, M. Arch, is a graduate student in Architectural Sciences at Laval University's School of Architecture in Quebec, Canada. Her thesis concerns the typological characterization and spatial syntax analysis of primary schools in Quebec, under the supervision of Carole Després and François Dufaux. She is an active member of the Groupe Interdisciplinaire sur les Banlieues (GIRBa) and participates in outreach activities and conferences.

Martin Maguire is a lecturer and Research Fellow at the Loughborough Design School. He studied Computer Science and Ergonomics (Loughborough) and has a PhD in Human-Computer Interaction (Leicester Polytechnic). He is a human factors researcher at Loughborough University and has worked on many projects in relation to inclusive design—kitchens to support independent living, home appliances, interactive kiosks and websites to enable their easier use by all. He has also been involved in a number of collaborative projects to develop usability requirements and evaluation methods for use within EU projects and internationally. His main areas of research and teaching are HCI, Usability, and User Experience Design for interactive systems.

Donald L. McEachron is a Teaching Professor and serves as Coordinator for Academic Assessment and Quality Improvement for the School of Biomedical Engineering, Science and Health Systems at Drexel University. Dr. McEachron holds a B.A. in

Behavioral Genetics from the University of California at Berkeley and a Ph.D. in Neuroscience from the University of California at San Diego. In December, 2006, he received a M.S. in Information Science from Drexel University. Dr. McEachron has published in numerous areas, including image processing, chronobiology, psychiatry, education and human evolution.

Susan O'Hara, PhD, MPH, RN is a post-doctoral faculty member and embedded scholar with the Schools of Nursing and Architecture at Clemson University's School of Health Research (CUSHR). Dr. O'Hara, served as the director of cardiopulmonary rehabilitation where she wrote the first hospital business plan to determine feasibility of building a new rehabilitation center in an adjoining community catchment area. This business plan was based on the triangulation of epidemiology, economic, and clinical care outcome data. She has also presented nationally at academic and trade conferences and has a strong record of peer reviewed publications. Her current ethnographic research interests are focused on Macrocognition in the Health Care Built Environment – how the layout of a space affects interprofessional adaptation of cognition to complexity and patient care quality and safety.

Neville Owen has a Ph.D. in experimental psychology. He is Head of the Behavioral Epidemiology Laboratory at the Baker Heart and Diabetes Institute in Melbourne, Australia, a National Health and Medical Research Council Senior Principal Research Fellow, and Distinguished Professor in Health Sciences at Swinburne University. His research deals with preventing type 2 diabetes, cardiovascular disease, and cancer through understanding and influencing physical inactivity and sedentary behaviors—too little exercise *and* too much sitting.

Jill Pable is a professor at Florida State University and a fellow and past national president of the Interior Design Educators Council. She holds B.S. and M.F.A. degrees in Interior Design and a Ph.D. degree in Instructional Technology. Her research focuses on the design of environments for the disadvantaged and is the originator of *Design Resources for Homelessness*, a research-informed online resource for architectural designers and service organizations creating facilities for homeless persons. She believes that design can make life more interesting, fulfilling, and humane.

A. Ray Pentecost III is the Director of the Center for Health Systems and Design in the College of Architecture at Texas A&M University and holds the Ronald L. Skaggs and Joseph G. Sprague Chair of Health Facilities Design. He is a registered Architect, Board Certified in the health care architecture specialty. He has been named a Fellow both in the American Institute of Architects (FAIA) and in the American College of Healthcare Architects (FACHA).

Denise Piché is associate professor at the Ecole d'architecture, Université Laval. She retired after 37 years as professor where she specialized in the domains of person-environment relationships, architectural programming, and urban design with a specific focus on health care, education, and aging. She is an active member of a multi-disciplinary research team on "Living in Northern Quebec", a partnership project with Canadian indigenous communities, and she remains active in long-term collaborations with institutions in Vietnam and Senegal.

Jon A. Sanford is a Professor and Director of the Center for Assistive Technology and Environmental Access in Georgia Tech's College of Design. He is also a co-Director of the Rehabilitation Engineering Research Center on Technologies for Successful Aging with Disability, supported by the Department of Health and Human Services. He is internationally recognized for his expertise in universal design and accessible housing and is the author of "Design for the Ages: Universal Design as a Rehabilitation Strategy".

Takemi Sugiyama's work focuses on built environment and active living. He has a Master of Architecture from Virginia Tech and a Ph.D. in Environment-Behaviour Studies from University of Sydney. After more than ten years of research experience in urban design and public health, he has recently joined the Institute for Health & Ageing, Australian Catholic University. He has published more than 70 peer-reviewed papers. He is a certified architect (Japan) and Associate Editor, Journal of Transport and Health.

Susan S. Szenasy is Publisher and Editor in Chief of *Metropolis*, the award-winning New York City-based magazine of architecture and design at all scales. Since 1986 she has lead the publication and its other media platforms through decades of landmark design journalism, achieving domestic and international recognition. She is a pioneer in connecting environmental stewardship with design, and a tireless advocate for human centered design. A book of her writings and talks, *Szenasy, Design Advocate*, was published in 2015 by Metropolis Books/DAP.

Ellen Taylor, Ph.D., AIA, MBA, EDAC, is the Vice President for Research at The Center for Health Design, where she leads multiple research initiatives focused on the relationship between the built environment and outcomes. She has a B.Arch from Cornell University, MBA degrees from Columbia University and London Business School, and a Ph.D. from Loughborough University in the UK. She serves on the Editorial Advisory Board of the Health Environments Research & Design (HERD) Journal.

Elif Tural, Ph.D., is an Assistant Professor of Interior Design in the School of Architecture + Design at Virginia Tech. Tural received her Ph.D. in Environmental Design and Planning from Arizona State University. She has a multi-disciplinary design background, including an MFA in Interior Architecture, and a B.Arch. Tural's research focuses on design factors for active and healthy living in senior residential environments and her teaching emphasizes the significance of evidence-based, socially- and environmentally-responsive design.

Lisa Waxman, Ph.D., is a professor and chair of the Department of Interior Architecture & Design at Florida State University. Her research addresses place and design for special populations. She holds an NCIDQ certificate, is a LEED-AP, and a licensed designer in Florida. Waxman is a past president and fellow of the Interior Design Educators Council and a member of the American Society of Interior Designers. She currently serves on the board of the Council for Interior Design Accreditation.

FOREWORD

In the summer of 2016, I served on an architecture awards jury; apparently I was chosen for a specific purpose. I was there as someone sensitive to interiors, usually a large category in these competitions. But, as I was told, last year's jurors had a hard time judging the category; one jury member even went so far as to say, it's not architecture. This, of course, leads me to ask, "What is architecture for, if not for the human beings who inhabit it?"

The book in your hands will clear up any confusion that may linger about architecture's most important role: human habitation. The form, the façade, the detailing are subservient to the spaces within: how interiors receive and manage natural light, flow into each other, aid the many and varied human functions therein, relate to the natural environments that may live on its roofs, facades, outcroppings, adjacent gardens, and walkways are all important to the health of the people who use these buildings.

This complex case for modern habitation is supported by research in the sciences, medicine, behavior, culture, policy—each documenting human concerns in an over-populated, rapidly urbanizing world. It is no surprise that health is at the center of this research. Whereas we used to talk about "sustainability," today we are certain that our stewardship of our natural environment is key to our well-being, our very survival. Our growing understanding of this reality is supported by the digital culture that connects us to people and their ideas about how to live lightly on the land, from every corner of the globe.

Some of these knowledge fields are in the midst of forming the ways of the twenty-first century. For instance, material health is undergoing a slow evolution, often offering unsatisfying answers to architects looking for toxin-free products. Government legislation—local, national, international—shows some signs of progress. Certainly, the daily missives that come across my computer screen from the EPA tell a hopeful story of the massive clean-up of poisoned swaths of earth and water, left in the wake of the industrial processes of the last century. Today corporate citizenship is on the side of upgrading manufacturing processes to where no refuse goes into landfills or seeps into groundwater or the rivers and brooks adjacent to the factories. At the same time, advocacy groups for clean and healthy materials are frustrated by the secrecy surrounding the material content of the products made at these factories, on the grounds that the mix of chemicals that make up materials—from furnishings to building products—are proprietary.

Aside from the complexity of our chemically infused materials, and the ongoing effort to reveal their molecular components, and redesign them to be as toxin free as possible, another monolithic approach is being dismantled: the evergreen topic of human habitation and the complexity of our species, hitherto the subject of philosophers, psychologists, novelists, artists, but only a few architects.

As we amend the modernist beliefs in pure rationalism, we begin to understand just how much of what makes us human has been ignored by those responsible for designing and constructing the built environment. Research, observation, and intuition reveal us to be creatures with a spiritual and emotional core, traits that twentieth-century architecture denied. Although there has been a lot of talk about our need for "messy vitality," our ever expanding building stock—always taller skyscrapers in every major city with seemingly little understanding of the climate, terrain, culture, material resources of the region in which they're built—continue to provide interior environments designed less for the people who inhabit them, and more for the financial bottom line of developers.

Whereas there has been much talk about "people centered design" for many years now, the idea is finally getting re-examined by businesses and institutions everywhere. As the generational shift is reshaping life patterns and behaviors, and as digital technology requires whole new ways of doing business, working, behaving, connecting, the value of a single human being is being reintroduced into conversations about the built environment.

Just think of how K-12 education has shifted into a new gear. Kids learn online, from books, by making things, by working with each other in small to large groups, guided by teachers as facilitators, not so much the sole authority figures of the twentieth-century classroom. Behaviors that assume mutual respect for well-earned knowledge, technical know-how, communication skills, critical thinking based on solid information, all contribute to a new valuation of educating a populace for the complexities of digital life in local/global cultures. These students make the most sought after employees of the twenty-first century.

In observing the architecture that supports these new workers, inside and outside, it's easy to see that these buildings and their outdoor environments are made for people with independent minds. Thus the twentieth-century's industrial model for workers—health care, education, workplace, retail—is challenged by their creative ideas, technical skills, respect of the environment, and the need to connect with community.

The fluid spaces provided for this valued worker emphasize the health and well-being of everyone in the organization. From serving fresh foods, to providing outdoor spaces and walkways for meetings, monastic retreats for heads-down work, and opportunities to exercise, these are deemed essential to building the businesses' bottom line. Productivity, that ever-elusive measurement of twentieth-century interiors, in a creative economy is measured by constant innovation. While "innovation" was the mantra of the last century, today it is seen as essential to the survival and prosperity of any institution, be it school, office, or healthy communities.

In fact, the old ways of building for highly segregated functions are being challenged by innovative companies of all kinds. For instance, the massive hospital complexes, still dominating much of health care, are seen as outmoded, often deadly incubators of super bugs, inhumane in their factory-like treatment of the ill and infirm. There's much talk about building healthy communities, in line with many of the mixed-use developments rising in dense urban environments everywhere.

The healthy community is seen as a lifelong commitment to fresh, local foods (some communities grow their own); a neighborhood kitchen and restaurant where neighbors can learn food preparation; opportunities for exercise that might include bike lanes, sidewalks, soccer fields, yoga classes; a neighborhood clinic with ties to a nearby hospital when needed; schools with outdoor classrooms and within walking distance from home; provision for jobs supported by maker spaces, we-work-like aggregations of small offices with communal spaces; and plenty of parks and green spaces in buildings and outside that expose everyone to the health benefits of sunlight.

The text you are about to read in *Health and Well-being for Interior Architecture* provides a detailed and smartly argued case for the humane environments that express the twenty-first-century ethos.

Susan S. Szenasy, Publisher & Editor in Chief,
Metropolis

1

TRADITIONAL AND ALTERNATIVE APPROACHES TO HEALTH AND WELL-BEING

Lynne M. Dearborn

Health and Well-being: Relations and Interactions

Public health policy and practice place substantial and increasing significance on environmental characteristics linked to health. Consequently, designers are poised to play a meaningful role confronting growing rates of physical and mental illness, merging their creativity with new scientific evidence linking health and well-being to many environmental elements that humans regularly encounter. Those who endorse the World Health Organization's expansive definition of health often lead contemporary global health initiatives. They move beyond a narrow biomedical view and interpret health as "a state of complete physical, mental, and social well-being."[1] Yet, conceptions of health and well-being and the environment's role in them still vary greatly around the world and among different professions. Designers must explore these conceptions and how they influence beliefs about the environment's role in improving quality of life if they are to bridge mind, body, and community through design to engender total physical, mental, and social well-being.

Health, assessed through instrumental measures of a body's state of physical repair, is only one component in scholarly conceptions of well-being.[2] Recent attention to well-being in several social science disciplines has spawned thoughtful discussions that interpret well-being as an all-inclusive, integrative mix of numerous objective and subjective considerations.[3] From design, the Interconnected Model of Well-Being[4] suggests the physical environment is not a neutral backdrop, instead influencing individual well-being in a holistic and integrative way, from the scale of the person to the community, through five dimensions of existence: spiritual, mental, emotional, social, and physical. Well-being can be operationalized "as a dynamic process and state of being . . . [enabling people to] sense how their lives are going, through the interaction between their circumstances [e.g., physical environment], activities and psychological resources or mental capacities."[5]

The five dimensions of existence noted above and the ways that each is linked to the environment may be interpreted differently depending on cultural background, professional orientation, and context. How we design to affect the physical, social, and psychological aspects of the environment to achieve good health and superior quality of life depends on recognizing that concepts of health and well-being inspire multiple meanings for people. The following discussion, using examples from diverse culture and lifestyle groups, illustrates myriad beliefs about health and well-being and the relationship of these to environmental considerations. It introduces a framework useful for designers and builders of the environment as they plan, accommodate, and promote health and well-being through their work.

Paradigms, Ontologies, and Epistemology

To interpret sometimes conflicting information and ideas encountered when seeking to promote health and well-being through environmental design, it is important to determine the paradigm under which any knowledge is considered "fact." A paradigm embodies a particular worldview, or set "of beliefs and assumptions that describe reality. . . a worldview provides the interpretive lens one uses to understand reality and one's existence within it."[6] One's worldview establishes the basic beliefs about "what is, what is important, and what ought to be."[7] While individuals in contemporary society may not consciously contemplate their worldview, each of us possesses an interpretive framework or description of the world that guides our perceptions and behaviors. This framework grows from individual experience and views shared with others who agree and operate under a similar worldview. Basic beliefs within a worldview are accepted solely on faith, and for those operating within the worldview are not open to question or testing.

Within and outside the scholarly realm, a vast array of worldviews and their associated assumptions about person-environment relationships guide conceptions of health and well-being. The worldview one embraces and functions within may be influenced by culture, for example, through beliefs about forces operating within the universe. Likewise, one's accepted paradigm or worldview may be influenced by professional or scholarly perspective. For example, a scholar within the sciences whose understanding of the universe is guided by an expectation that the world can be objectively studied, gleans "facts" through quantification, prediction, and statistical formulae. While it may reside in the subconscious, one's worldview defines two important characteristics, ontology and epistemology, that guide thinking and behavior as well as ideas about health and well-being. Personal ontology dictates one's understanding of the nature of being, the kinds of things that have existence,[8] and therefore what can affect health and well-being, and what it is possible to know about those influences. Personal epistemology follows directly from personal ontology;[9] it dictates the relationship between the individual and the forces influencing them and what can be ascertained about those forces. Epistemology concerns how individuals may go about studying and comprehending ontology. Thus, for one interested in conducting research on health, well-being, and environment, data collection methods follow directly from one's epistemology. A range of worldviews currently inform thinking in various global locations; these illustrate the diverse ways that ontologies contribute to different understandings of the health–well-being–environment triad.

Worldviews, Ontologies and Well-being: Environment Linkages

Metaphysical assumptions about how the universe works underpin beliefs about what makes us sick, what keeps us well, and what conditions in the environment promote well-being, helping us to achieve optimal daily and long-term function and overall life satisfaction. The major characteristic distinguishing the two primary worldview categories influencing contemporary health-related practice, or health-belief system, is whether or not the practice is grounded in the scientific method.[10] Thus, the following is divided into two main discussions. The first explores contemporary "Western" medicine's evidence-based worldview that addresses illness through hypothesis-testing and positive theory, refined by systematic observation, measurement, and deductive reasoning. The second discusses medical systems considered by "Western" medicine as alternative and complementary, including a range of "traditional" or culture-informed medical systems as well as alternative "modern" systems. The short overview and several illustrations elucidating underlying worldviews and practices are not exhaustive but provide stimuli for thought on the diverse definitions of health and well-being, and the environment's role in them.

Worldviews Rooted in the Scientific Method

The most widely held worldview regarding health within much of the developed world underpins evidence-based practice. Health care conducted within this worldview is labeled conventional, Western, mainstream, or allopathic medicine. It is practiced by individuals who have earned M.D. (Doctor of Medicine) or D.O. (Doctor of Osteopathy) degrees as well as allied health professionals such as registered nurses, physical therapists, and psychologists.[11] Associated with conventional medicine, public health seeks to assure societal conditions within which people remain free of illness.[12]

Evidence-based health practice originates from early systematic investigations, before which many healers believed that illness resulted from divine acts or an imbalance of humors.[13] James Lind's 1746 application of a series of possible treatments for scurvy to pairs of Scottish sailors contributed to a new paradigm of health practice and identified regular doses of lime juice as the best means for preventing scurvy among sailors. This demonstrates one of several early contributions to conventional medicine's foundation.[14] Over the intervening 270 years, the scientific method has been applied to health-based research.[15] Today, conventional medicine is distinguished by therapies and treatments that apply "scientifically proven, evidence-based medicine supported by solid data."[16] Conventional treatments garnered 96 percent of U.S. medical spending in 2012,[17] suggesting a strong belief in its efficacy.

Contemporary public health shares this worldview anchored in the scientific method. Empirical evidence that supports public health practice includes "ongoing systematic collection, analysis, and interpretation of data essential to the planning, implementation, and evaluation of public health," incorporating community-scale demographics, morbidity and mortality data, and disease incidence and prevalence.[18] Epidemiology, which studies the incidence, distribution, and control of disease in a population,[19] provides an important foundation for public health. Public health includes a sub-discipline, environmental health, focused on promoting healthy environments and controlling environmental hazards detrimental to the public's health.[20]

The adverse living and working conditions generated by the Industrial Revolution contributed to high mortality rates, particularly among residents who were poor or working-class, prompting development of the public and environmental health professions.[21] Quantitative measures of population health, combined with systematic observations of environmental conditions and exposures, enabled scientists (e.g., John Snow) to establish links between specific diseases, such as cholera, and environmental conditions. Thus, within the worldview informed by the scientific method, health, but more so illness, is something that can and must be systematically and objectively observed and quantified. Conditions in the environment are likewise observed and quantified. These quantitative data are analyzed statistically to determine relationships between environmental conditions and health outcomes.

Historically, practices allied with conventional medicine, including public and environmental health, have focused on studying and treating specific causes of illness as opposed to promoting general well-being and wellness. These efforts yielded an average 30-year lifespan increase for Americans during the twentieth century.[22] However, current chronic disease trends and their convergence with particular environmental conditions have recently prompted new wellness initiatives in public and environmental health.

Complementary and Alternative Medical Worldviews

Conventional medicine's literature labels a diverse body of medical, health care, wellness, and well-being beliefs, products, and practices originating outside the Western evidence-based system as complementary and alternative medicine (CAM).[23] Complementary practices are used in conjunction with conventional therapies while alternative practices replace conventional medical care. Over 45 percent of U.S. residents used CAM during 2012,[24] spending 34 billion dollars.[25] CAM practices represent a range of worldviews. What links them is their belief in something other than hypotheses tested and retested through systematic, objective study. However, studies employing the scientific method have been used to test the efficacy of some CAM practices and a number of these have been integrated into conventional medicine over time.[26]

People of diverse backgrounds use CAM for a range of reasons.[27] In the U.S., usage is higher among women, adults with higher incomes and advanced levels of education, and among Native Americans.[28] CAM is most frequently used by those with chronic, recurrent, or serious illness such as HIV infection, rheumatoid arthritis, and cancer.[29] CAM use in the U.S. grows from its perceived underlying optimism and personal attention;[30] its self-help approach;[31] the appeal of treatments perceived as less harmful than conventional medicine because they are "natural" or "less invasive;"[32] greater awareness of cultures that typically use CAM;[33] suspicion of and dissatisfaction with the conventional health care system;[34] and an increasing appreciation that many things contribute to health and well-being.[35] A commonly accepted taxonomy identifies three CAM types: mind-body practices, traditional medical systems, and "modern" medical systems.[36] Mind-body practices are based in either traditional medical systems or alternative "modern" medical systems, a categorization that frames the following discussion comparing two worldviews types underlying alternative medicine.

Culture-informed Worldviews of Traditional Medical Systems

Traditional medical systems provide holistic mind-body conceptions of health, illness preventions, and cures; they are closely linked to the prevailing worldview of the culture within which they exist.[37] These belief systems not only explain human problems and treatment rationales but also support other culturally embedded ethical and social norms in response to conceptions of the common good. The health of an individual is incomprehensible outside the context of "his or her community, natural environment and spirit world."[38] Cultural worldviews are often rooted in specific cosmologies, creation myths, or geomantic beliefs about otherworldly forces operating within the universe that can be divined through interpretation of figures or geographic features. Ill-health and misfortune are generally thought to result from an imbalance of natural elements or life-force, an improper flow of energy, or conflict between the human and spirit worlds. These traditions often emphasize prevention by maintaining "proper" relations between individuals and their community; appropriate acknowledgement, response to, and respect for the natural environment, its forces, and embedded spirits; and fitting appeasement and respect for the spirit world. Individuals with particular gifts, often naturally endowed, are able to read the forces in the natural world, feel the power imbalances in a community, or "transcend the normal state of being and communicate with the spirit world on behalf of their communities."[39]

Myriad traditional medical systems exist in various cultural contexts around the world, often coexisting alongside Western biomedicine,[40] but as these systems address the integrated mind-body and what the Western scientific worldview labels mystical or supernatural,[41] they are often categorized as religious or spiritual as distinct from medical. Two systems, increasingly well known around the world, are the Chinese *qi*-based system and *Ayurveda*, a system rooted in Hinduism.[42] The Hmong, a cultural group with history in southern China and Southeast Asia, practice a system of traditional medicine that, while distinctly Hmong, resembles the Chinese system.[43]

Three identifiable but interwoven components comprise Hmong traditional practice: spiritual beliefs (animism and ancestor worship), geomantic beliefs, and herbalism.[44] As animists, Hmong believe that both living and inanimate objects contain spirits and/or souls and also that supernatural beings are involved in every aspect of life. The most crucial are the human–world/spirit–world relationships apparent in birth, death, and sickness.[45] The Hmong believe that a person has three *plig* (souls) that separate at death: one soul passes to heaven, one soul to the grave, and one re-embodies through reincarnation within one's clan.[46] For the Hmong, illness and misfortune result when the spirits of dead relatives are not satisfied, when one's *plig* has been stolen, or when someone directs evil spirits to cause harm.[47] Shaman (*txiv neeb*) "see" and communicate with the spirit world and thus are consulted in the event of illness or misfortune.[48] Traditionally, Hmong believe that spirits inhabit a house: patrilineal ancestor spirits, the spirit of the cooking hearth, the spirit of the ritual hearth, the door spirit, specific bedroom spirits, and spirits of wealth and richness who protect household members.[49]

Spirits inhabit altars opposite the main door; these are often connected to the door head by an ensemble of cloth or strings to facilitate the spirits' path, as Figure 1.1 shows.[50]

New houses in a village should not obstruct the clear, straight path that spirits take to enter the front door.[51] Even among immigrant Hmong, annual ceremonies and rituals are performed to feed ancestor spirits, to call the soul of an ill person

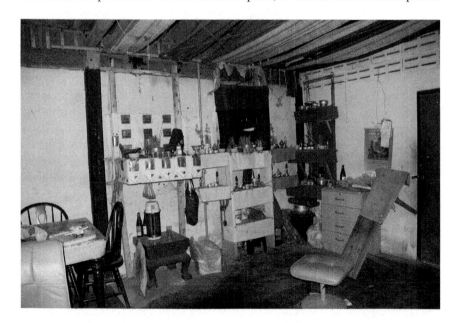

FIGURE 1.1   Household Altars Opposite Front Door: Prosperity Altar Left, Shaman's Altar Right (Khun Klang, Thailand)

or a newborn, and for otherworldly communications.[52] Many Christian Hmong in Southeast Asia and the U.S. combine traditional practices and Western medicine to appease watchful spirits and address illness.[53]

Hmong residential choice is influenced by geomantic beliefs. Labeled *loojmen*, these beliefs provides rules for siting villages, houses, and the graves of ancestors according to the contours of the mountains and watercourses formed in mountain valleys.[54] Just as incorrectly sited graves and houses bring illness and adversity to occupants, villages contradicting *loojmen* principles inevitably bring misfortune for inhabitants.[55] Traditionally, villages and houses were auspiciously sited to harmonize with surrounding geography and respond to the natural geography's "currents of breath" dictated by *loojmen*.[56] The importance of the geomantic worldview for health and well-being of Southeast Asian Hmong is relatively well documented yet little studied among U.S. Hmong immigrants.[57]

The shaman who communicate with the spirit world are believed naturally gifted with their abilities; however, herbalism is practiced more widely by Hmong women who carry, "an enormous store of knowledge about (wild and cultivated) plants and the ailments for which they are useful" and pass this knowledge and the "spirit of medicine" to the next generation.[58] Herbal remedies may precede or complement shamanic treatment depending on the length and severity of the ailment and the perceived need to communicate with the spirit world for the cure.[59]

These three interwoven components of Hmong traditional practice link to and influence human relationships to the environment in various ways. The Hmong traditional medicine system is just one example of how such systems tie cultural worldviews with environment. Traditional medical systems often address forces within nature that influence the balance of bodily elements/energies and also individual forces that address otherworldly sprits.[60] Likewise, "Modern" Alternative Medicine usually responds to both individual and spiritual forces.

"Modern" Alternative Medical Worldviews

Many contemporary or "modern" alternative medical belief systems originated in the early 1800s in the U.S. and Europe. These systems are distinguishable from culture-informed worldviews of traditional medicine systems, discussed above, through professionalization built upon: established schools for training the next generation of healers, a common base of accepted theory and standardized treatments, and organized professional societies or published journals.[61] While distinct from each other in theoretical bases and accepted therapies, these "modern" alternative medical systems share a distinguishing worldview characteristic: the belief in "*vis medicatrix naturae*—the healing power of nature," whereby treatment should be based upon, "reparative powers of the body" and supported through natural means.[62] Many of these nature-based belief systems gained initial acceptance in the era when orthodox physicians used toxic drugs and invasive practices (e.g., bloodletting) as treatments with little scientific basis.[63] These treatments nonetheless provided heroic indications of the art of medicine and also distinguished orthodox from naturalistic healers.[64] Ontologically, nature-based worldviews believe that nature is a prime component of prevention and provides the most effective therapy, and often subscribe to a mind-body holism that is tied to an ideal lifestyle.[65]

Practitioners of alternative medicine diverge epistemologically from conventional medicine's beliefs that the root causes of illness and thus cures can be identified by anyone asking theory-derived questions of objectively collected data, and applying scientific methods. Conversely, therapies within nature-based alternative medicine are generally discovered intuitively and revealed to those who have a talent for connecting with and understanding nature and natural processes. In large part, "alternative medicine has followed an alternative science. . . [based in] intuition, common sense, patience, and close observation" rather than complex thinking and widespread experimentation.[66] Throughout the history of modern alternative medicine, its practitioners often have been conceived as healers who have the ability to return people to spiritual, psychological, emotional, and physical health.[67] These holistic, nature-based ideas of healing and well-being suggest that modern alternative medical belief systems conceptualize people, person-environment relations, and therapy in ways that are fundamentally different from those of conventional medicine but akin to culture-informed traditional systems.

Naturopathic medicine, one modern alternative medical system, is defined by its grounding in the nature-based worldview. The foundational principles of contemporary naturopathic medicine are: the healing power of nature, identify and treat the causes, doctor as teacher, treat the whole person, and prevention.[68] This medical system grows from health treatments conceived in the 1850s by German priest Sebastian Kneipp, and brought to the U.S. in the 1890s by Benedict Lust, who, after being restored to health through its treatments, was convinced that lives in America would be improved by broader access to the Kneippism's health treatments.[69]

In developing naturopathic practice, Lust added drugless therapies (e.g., natural diet, exercise in nature, sunbathing), and mental and spiritual healing through a moral lifestyle (based in biblical teaching) to Kneippism's treatments of hot, cold, and steam bathing, botanical and herbal extracts and teas administered through warm baths and orally, "hardening" to restore primitive vigor by frequent immersions in cold water and ninety-minute barefoot walks in the snow or wet grass.[70] He later augmented these with hardening therapies employing special health equipment and health clothing seeking to counter the then prevalently hypothesized softening attendant with urban life and environments. Lust contributed to naturopathy's professionalization at the turn of the twentieth century by establishing a monthly naturopathy periodical, the Naturopathic Society of America, and the American School of Naturopathy in New York City.[71]

Although the use of naturopathic medicine declined following Lust's death in 1945, it regained popularity in the 1960s and remains a prominent alternative medical system. Twenty states and territorial areas and five Canadian provinces currently have licensing or regulatory laws for naturopathic doctors (NDs) with 5,000 licensed NDs overall in those areas.[72] Naturopathic doctors treat the whole person by seeking to identify the cause of illness through understanding spirit, mind, and body. They place an emphasis on preventing ill-health through wellness and patient education, striving to support the body's own healing by empowering people to modify lifestyle, diet, and behavior and to become more spiritually aware. Treatments engage patients in the healing process through spiritual and lifestyle changes, and by employing natural substances such as herbal medicines and techniques like hydrotherapy, massage, and natural detoxification.[73]

Conclusions

The preceding discussion clarified two important points with respect to ongoing discussions of the relationships between the environment and health. First, it showed that biomedicine is only one of many ways to understand and interpret the person-heath-environment nexus. While development of the positivistic science of biomedicine capitalized on the trend toward rationalism that followed the Enlightenment, it ignored subjective and sensory reflection of contextual lived-experience.[74] Biomedicine's focus and privileging of what objectively can be measured with respect to a body's state of physical repair falls short of a framework that can support well-being and promote human wellness. Second, it showed that alternative medical belief systems conceptualize an inseparable mind-body-environment with implications for the built world's construction. Much can be learned from worldviews that underpin alternative and complementary medical belief systems and just as Western medicine has verified the efficacy of some alternative therapies so might these alternative medical belief systems offer ideas to be tested through health/well-being outcomes of environmental design.

If designers hope to create environments that support a more wholly satisfying existence, they must moderate total alliance with biomedicine and its conceptualization of the body as a physical machine disconnected from soul, spirit, or mind. Combining aspects of Western and alternative medical worldviews provides a basis for a comprehensive framework wherein a holistic state of well-being is possible. The framework proposed in Figure 1.2 conceptualizes individual well-being as nourished by mental, spiritual, emotional, occupational, physical, and social conditions of lived experience.

The environment is ever-present and supportive of each of these six dimensions of well-being and appropriate environmental design and construction is instrumental. When the environment supports our accomplishment of satisfying tasks, and promotes happiness and contentment, it contributes to our mental well-being. Environments that invoke a sense of awe remind us of the presence of a higher power, prompt our inner peace, and nourish our spiritual well-being. Environments appealing to our multiple senses contribute to the emotional dimension of well-being. Those that provide for our ambitions and nourish our need to be useful and creative, reinforce our occupational well-being. Our physical well-being is underpinned by environments that positively stimulate and support the needs of our physical bodies. Environments that engender positive feelings of ties to other humans and living creatures reinforce the social dimension of well-being.

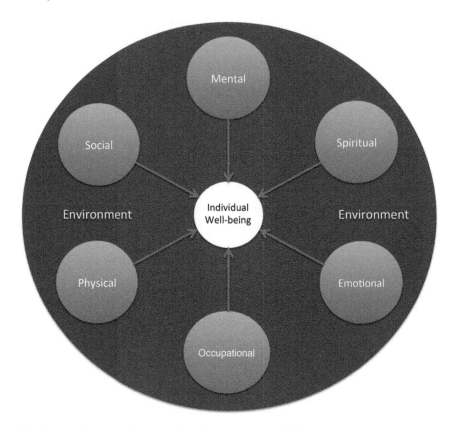

FIGURE 1.2 Dynamic Framework of Environmental Well-being

Well-being is a multi-dimensional, integrative, and all-encompassing condition that can be understood and achieved within the context of a worldview that acknowledges the inseparability of mind, body, and environment. Well-being combines mind and body wellness in equal measures and relies on built and natural environments that encourage us to think and act on those aspects of life that fulfill our human needs, appeal to our senses, and to our creativity.

Notes

1 WHO (World Health Organization), "WHO Definition of Health," www.who.int/about/definition/en/print.html.
2 Lindsay Sowman, "Towards a Landscape of Well-Being," in *Landscape, Well-Being and Environments*, eds. Richard Coles and Zoë Millman (Abingdon, Oxon: Routledge, 2013), 58–59.
3 Martin Seligman, *Flourish* (New York: Free Press, 2012), 5–8; Sebastien Fleuret and Sarah Atkinson, "Well-Being, Health and Geography," *New Zealand Geographer* 63, no. 3 (2007): 113.
4 Sara Warber, Katherine Irvine, Patrick Devine-Wright, and Kevin Gaston, "Modelling Well-Being and the Relationship Between Individuals and Their Environments," in

Landscape, Well-Being and Environments, eds. Richard Coles and Zoë Millman (Abingdon, Oxon: Routledge, 2013), 31.

5   Sowman, "Well-Being," 59.

6   Mark E. Koltko-Rivera, "The Psychology of Worldviews," *Review of General Psychology* 8, no. 1 (2004): 3.

7   Kathryn A. Johnson, Eric D. Hill, and Adam B. Cohen, "Integrating the Study of Culture and Religion: Toward a Psychology of Worldview," *Social and Personality Psychology Compass* 5, no. 3 (2011): 138.

8   Ibid.

9   Ibid., 146–147.

10 Sally Thorne, "Health Belief Systems in Perspective," *Journal of Advanced Nursing* 18, no. 12 (1993): 1931–1932.

11 MedicineNet, "Definition of Conventional Medicine," MedicineNet Inc., www.medicine net.com/script/main/art.asp?articlekey=33527.

12 Howard Frumkin, Arthur M. Wendel, Robin F. Abrams, and Emil Malizia, "An Introduction to Healthy Places," in *Making Healthy Places*, eds. Andrew L. Dannenberg, Howard Frumkin, and Richard J. Jackson (Washington, DC: Island Press, 2011), 6.

13 Paul A. Offit, *Do You Believe in Magic?* (New York: HarperCollins, 2013), 28.

14 Ibid., 30–31.

15 Linda Barnes, "Spirituality and Religion in Health Care," in *Cross-Cultural Medicine*, ed. Judyann Bigby (Philadelphia, PA: American College of Physicians, 2003), 237.

16 Phil B. Fontanarosa and George D. Lundberg, "Alternative Medicine Meets Science," *Journal of the American Medical Association* 280, no. 18 (1998): 1618.

17 Dan Munro, "U.S. Annual Healthcare Spending Is a Stunning $3.4 Trillion, Says Study," *Forbes / Pharma & Healthcare*, www.forbes.com/sites/danmunro/2014/11/17/new-deloitte-study-u-s-healthcare-spending-for-2012-was-over-3-4-trillion/#38a091b55ce8.

18 Frumkin, "Healthy Places," 14.

19 Merriam-Webster, "Epidemiology," Merriam-Webster, Inc., www.merriam-webster. com/dictionary/epidemiology.

20 Frumkin, "Healthy Places," 6.

21 Esther Sternberg, *Healing Spaces* (Cambridge: Belknap Press, 2009), 261.

22 Offit, *Believe in Magic*, 32.

23 Josephine P. Briggs, Dan L. Longo, Anthony S. Fauci, Dennis L. Kasper, Stephen L. Hauser, J. Larry Jameson, and Joseph Loscalzo, "Complementary, Alternative, and Integrative Health Practices," in *Harrison's Principles of Internal Medicine*, eds. Dennis L. Kasper et al. (New York: McGraw-Hill Medical, 2014), 14e-1.

24 Two analyses released in 2015 by the National Center for Complementary and Integrative Health showed that 11.6 percent of Americans ages 4–17 and 34 percent of adults used some type of complementary or alternative approach in 2012; see https://nccih. nih.gov/research/statistics/NHIS/bibliography.

25 Offit, *Believe in Magic*, 1.

26 C. Lee Ventola, "Current Issues Regarding Complementary and Alternative Medicine in the United States," *Pharmacy and Therapeutics* 35, no. 8 (2010): 462; Briggs, "Health Practices," 14e-3. One-quarter of modern plant-derived pharmaceuticals, with some basis in traditional practices, and the Lamaze Method of childbirth are among these.

27 Barnes, "Spirituality," 246.

28 Ventola, "Current Issues," 462.

29 Ibid., 463.

30 Briggs, "Health Practices," 14e-4.

31 Ibid.; Offit, *Believe in Magic*, 43.

32 Ibid.

33 Barnes, "Spirituality," 243; Ventola, "Current Issues," 465.

34 Ibid.

35 Ibid.

36 Briggs, "Health Practices," 14e-1.

37 Thorne, "Belief Systems," 1933.
38 Ibid., 1934.
39 Ibid., 1936.
40 Barnes, "Spirituality," 246.
41 Ibid., 249, 251.
42 Ibid., 248.
43 Nicholas Tapp, "Hmong Religion," *Asian Folklore Studies* 48 (1989): 59.
44 Robert Cooper, ed. *The Hmong* (Singapore: Times Edition Pte. Ltd., 1998), 103, 111–112.
45 Patricia V. Symonds, *Calling the Soul* (Seattle, WA: University of Washington Press, 2004), 11; Tapp, "Hmong," 59.
46 Symonds, *Calling*, 21.
47 Cooper, *Hmong*, 127–130.
48 Ibid., 127; Symonds, *Calling*, 12, 22.
49 Cooper, *Hmong*, 28; Symonds, *Calling*, 13.
50 Symonds, *Calling*, 13–16. Symonds describes Hmong altars in detail.
51 Cooper, *Hmong*, 31.
52 Jo Ann Koltyk, *New Pioneers in the Heartland* (Boston, MA: Allyn & Bacon, 1998), 119.
53 Cooper, *Hmong*, 135; Koltyk, *Pioneers*, 64–72. Koltyk discusses health beliefs and practices of immigrant Hmong.
54 Nicholas Tapp, "Geomancy and Development," *Ethnos* 53, no. 3–4 (1988): 230.
55 Ibid., 228.
56 Symonds, *Calling*, 12; Tapp, "Geomancy," 229; Cooper, *Hmong*, 30, 43.
57 Donald A. Ranard, "The Refugees and Their Carolina Roots," *The Washington Post*, November 29, 1986, www.washingtonpost.com/archive/lifestyle/1986/11/29/the-refu gees-and-their-carolina-roots/cddb1922-699c-4736-b571-e29070035c06/. Ranard provides one of the only descriptions of how geomantic beliefs influence ideal house placement for U.S.-immigrant Hmong.
58 Cooper, *Hmong*, 112.
59 Ibid.
60 Thorne, "Belief Systems," 1937.
61 James C. Whorton, *Nature Cures* (New York: Oxford University Press, 2002), 8.
62 Ibid., 6.
63 Whorton, *Nature*, 4–5; Arthur Wrobel, "Introduction," in *Pseudo-Science and Society in Nineteenth-Century America*, ed. Arthur Wrobel (Lexington: University Press of Kentucky, 1987), 4.
64 Whorton, *Nature*, 7.
65 Whorton, *Nature*, xii; Wrobel, *Pseudo-Science*, 6.
66 Whorton, *Nature*, 11.
67 Ibid.
68 Naturopathic Physicians, "House of Delegates Position Paper: Definition of Naturopathic Medicine," American Association of Naturopathic Physicians, www.naturopathic. org/content.asp?contentid=59.
69 Ibid.
70 Ibid., 198–199.
71 Steven D. Ehrlich, "Naturopathy," Univeristy of Maryland Medical Center, https:// umm.edu/health/medical/altmed/treatment/naturopathy; Whorton, *Nature*, 194.
72 Naturopathic Doctor Licensure, Association of Accredited Naturopathic Mecial Colleges, https://aanmc.org/resources/licensure/.
73 Sophie Hill, Alan Bensoussan, Stephen P. Myers, Jo Condron, and Song Mei Wu, "Consumers of Naturopathy and Western Herbal Medicine," in *The Practice and Regulatory Requirements of Naturopathy and Western Herbal Medicine*, eds. Vivian Lin et al. (Melbourne: La Trobe University, 2005), 243.
74 Thorne, "Belief Systems," 1932.

2

CO-PRODUCING OUR HABITAT FOR HEALTH AND WELL-BEING

Roderick J. Lawrence

Introduction

Our living environments are complex with many material and non-physical components that extend from the housing unit in which we live, to the location of the street and neighborhood, and the city and region beyond our immediate surroundings. These units of analysis and understanding are inscribed in ecological and geo-political levels that extend to a global or international level.[1]

Health is multi-dimensional because it includes genetics, tangible biophysical dimensions and neuropsychological dimensions. The multiple relations between the residential environment in which we live and our health are a complex web of interconnections (see Table 2.1). It is possible to determine whether housing conditions influence the health of occupants and how the health of individuals can influence her/his housing conditions. For example, housing conditions, and homelessness, are key components in the chain of explanatory factors linking poverty and inequality to the health status of individuals and households.[2]

The relationships between housing and health ought to be considered in terms of the multiple factors that influence human habitats and health status, and the interrelations between them. An ecological perspective recognizes that behavioral, biological, cultural, economic, social, physical and political factors need to be considered if a broad, comprehensive understanding is to complement disciplinary and sector-based interpretations.[3] In order to integrate these dimensions, it is necessary to go beyond interpretations that rely solely on the biomedical model of health. Transdisciplinary and collaborative research contributions involving different disciplines and professions are necessary. They should adopt a holistic interpretation that rejects any kind of single causal statistical interpretation.[4] They need to consider the interrelations between multiple factors in the societal context in which they occur.

This author argues for a shift from traditional disciplinary and professional approaches to interdisciplinary and transdisciplinary research and professional practice.[5] Hopefully, these kinds of collaborative contributions will serve as a catalyst for many more innovative projects that promote health and quality of life in the future.

Interpretations of Health and Well-being

The word health is derived from the old English word "hal" meaning whole, healed and sound. Health is a difficult concept to define and has been interpreted in diverse ways. Nonetheless, health has intrinsic value that cannot be quantified only in monetary units. Health is fundamentally different from other attributes of life owing to the unique status of the human body. Unlike other objects, the body is possessed by an individual that constitutes the person; there is no such thing as a disembodied person. Each person may be a consumer of, and an object to which health services are directed. Simultaneously, each person is an active producer of her/his health by following habits of diet, exercise and hygiene, and other lifestyle traits, which may or may not be conducive to health promotion.

Health

The definition of the World Health Organization states that health is "not merely the absence of disease and infirmity but a state of optimal physical, mental and social well-being."[6] This definition is idealistic, but it has the merit of not focusing on illness and disease, which have often been considered as either temporary or permanent impairment, or the malfunctioning of a single or several constituents of the human body. Given that the World Health Organization's definition of health includes social well-being, then the most common interpretations of health ought to be enlarged. The World Health Organization also states that the enjoyment of the highest attainable standard of health is one of the fundamental rights of every person without distinction of race, religion, political, economic or social condition.

Health is defined in this chapter as a condition resulting from the interrelations between humans and their biological, chemical, economic, physical and social environment. These components of human habitats, shown in Table 2.1, should be compatible with basic needs and full functional activity including biological reproduction.[7] Health is the result of direct pathological effects of chemicals, some biological agents and radiation and the influence of physical, psychological and social dimensions of daily life including housing, transport and other characteristics of metropolitan areas. For example, improved access to medical services is a common characteristic of urban neighborhoods that is rare in rural areas.

In the field of health promotion, health is not considered as an abstract condition. It is the ability of an individual to achieve her/his potential and to respond positively to the challenges of daily life. Health is an asset or a resource for everyday life rather than a standard or goal that ought to be achieved.[8] This interpretation is pertinent for studies of the interrelations between health, human behavior and built environments because the environmental and social conditions in specific localities influence human relations, may induce stress and can have positive or negative impacts on the health status of groups and individuals. This implies that the capacity of the health sector to deal with health promotion and prevention is limited and that close collaboration with other sectors would be beneficial and necessary to improve health status. It is crucial to pose the question *how* architectural and urban designs can positively influence health.[9] In essence, there is a fundamental shift from the question whether buildings, public spaces and urban neighborhoods can make people ill, to a new question about how housing, buildings and planning can promote health and a quality of life.

During the last four decades a growing number of contributions from around the world have translated those positive factors that promote human health and well-being. For example, some architects and designers have been working on the design of health care buildings, schools and office buildings following a salutogenic interpretation using the introduction of indoor vegetation and/or views to natural landscapes.[10]

Well-being

Well-being is a contested concept without consensus, based on social and cultural representations. Well-being is considered to be a positive, evolutionary and multi-dimensional state with objective and subjective components (hedonic and eudemonic well-being) and measurements.[11] It is important to consider the interrelated dimensions of health and well-being: cultural, economic, psychological, physical and social. Each of these dimensions could be influenced positively by the design and use of buildings and public spaces.[12] Mental health is defined as a state of well-being in which every individual realizes his or her own potential, can cope with the normal stresses of life, can work productively and fruitfully and is able to make a contribution to her/his community.

Environment

The environment of any living species is multi-dimensional and complex.[13] Therefore, residential environments should not be interpreted as a neutral background for human behavior as it frequently has been in environmental psychology. The human ecology perspective applied in this chapter interprets the processes, patterns, products and mediating factors that regulate human behavior in residential environments using a systemic framework explained by Rob Dyball and Barry Newell.[14] A dialectical and integrated approach is necessary to overcome the chasm between those health professionals who blame the environmental conditions for the incidence of ill-health, those environmental activists who blame local firms and national and multinational companies for the deplorable state of the environment and those architects, housing administrators and urban planners who still do not

TABLE 2.1   The interrelationships between housing conditions and health status are multiple and this representation is developed as a conceptual reference framework. (The numbers in parentheses are explained in the table footnotes. Thanks to Mr. Matthias Braubach, WHO European Office, Bonn, Germany for comments on a preliminary version)

THE RESIDENTIAL CONTEXT OF HEALTH

Scale / Factors	Physical / Material	Social, Political & Economic	Psychological / Cultural
Individual **Family**	Personal traits, Personal space, Lifestyle (1)	Income, Social class, Profession (6)	Meaning of housing, Autonomy, Meaning of health (11)
Household	Quality of Dwelling, Lifestyle (2)	Tenure security, Household traits (7)	Meaning of family, Neighbors/ Privacy (12)
Neighborhood **City/Region**	Environmental conditions, Infrastructure (3)	Accessibility and affordability of health and social services (8)	Community life, Social capital, Sense of security (13)
National **Continent**	Housing regulations, Health services (4)	Housing, health and social policies (9)	Diversity of lifestyles, Housing diversity (14)
Global	Climate change, Ozone layer (5)	Globalization, Peace, conflicts (10)	Population mobility, Refugees (15)

(1) The physical/material characteristics of the individual include his/her personal space, lifestyle and personal traits (age, gender etc.) that may prescribe the functional use of the residential environment. The individual can be one person in a household of several residents but in developed countries the share of one person households is high and increasing.

(2) Housing quality includes quantifiable and qualitative dimensions of the housing unit and its immediate surroundings such as the area and volume of space for each household, the characteristics of the physical fabric (indoor and outdoor air quality, damp, mold, hot/cold seasonal temperatures, noise and the quality of equipment in kitchen and bathrooms etc.).

(3) The environmental conditions of residential neighborhoods include ambient air quality, noise, soil and water quality, whereas infrastructure refers to the supply of potable water, sewage disposal, collection and treatment of solid and liquid wastes, site drainage, supplies of energy and access to public green spaces and other facilities.

(4) Physical and material characteristics of residential buildings and environmental conditions can be prescribed by national housing regulations, building construction standards and environmental laws. Likewise the quality and quantity of health and social services in local communities is related to national policies and funding.

(5) Climate change and the depletion of the ozone layer are global concerns which have impacts on residential environments and human health owing to erratic weather patterns (storms, flooding, frosts, heat waves) as well as the propagation of vectors diseases.

(6) The income of an individual and household is crucial for access to suitable housing and health care. Income, profession and security of employment are crucial indicators of individual and household poverty, housing conditions and access to health and social services.

(7) Security of housing tenure especially in the formal rental sector and informal housing is crucial for low-income households including one-parent families, migrants, unemployed persons and elderly residents in need of heath care and social services.

(8) Social and health services may or may not be located in residential neighborhoods. Public transportation or mobile service units may reduce the distance to these services. However, accessibility should not be isolated from the affordability of health care and social services for low-income residents.

(9) The accessibility and affordability of housing, health and social services are influenced by national policies that may promote the public or private sector. Governments may or may not subsidize medical and welfare services especially of individuals and households in need.

(10) Globalization policies have influenced housing markets, access to jobs and also a wide range of production and consumption patterns, especially food available in local supermarkets. Ethnic, religious and other conflicts occur in all regions of the world and influence living and working conditions as well as health.

(11) The meaning of housing, like the meaning of health, varies between individuals and social groups in the same society as well as between cultures. In contrast to dependency, the autonomy of the resident is a crucial psychological dimension of housing and health.

(12) Household and family bonding, neighbor relations and the immediate social environment are crucial components of residential environments that help define a sense of privacy identity, belonging and self-esteem, which are associated with residential satisfaction.

(13) Residents may be strongly integrated or isolated from local associations and community life and this can influence the degree of mutual aid, a sense of security and help them meet the challenge of difficult housing and health situations in specific neighborhoods.

(14) Diverse housing styles and lifestyles have always existed but this has been accentuated by the mass media and tourism. Often, imported types of housing construction and consumer goods (including clothing and food) are inappropriate for local climatic conditions and may clash with traditional societal values.

(15) Population and residential mobility is increasing in many countries. The homelessness of refugees due to conflicts or war is a major humanitarian concern that impacts on local housing and job markets. Climate or environmental refugees are expected to increase rapidly during the twenty-first century.

Source: Created by Roderick Lawrence.

accept the reciprocal relationship between people and environment at the small scale of the housing unit and neighborhood, or at larger geo-political scales.

Residential Environment

Housing is meant to address basic human needs for shelter and security by providing protection against climatic conditions (excessive heat and cold) and unwanted intrusions from insects, rodents and environmental nuisances, such as noise, that may be harmful for health and well-being. Housing contains household activities and possessions. Forty years ago John Turner made the important distinction between housing as a noun and housing as a verb.[15] According to Turner, housing can be considered as a product (from an individual housing unit to the housing stock in a neighborhood or city). He also suggested that housing can be considered as a process by the provision and maintenance of all kinds of residential buildings either by public authorities or private initiatives. Turner's interpretation of housing enables researchers and practitioners to consider the multiple interrelations between housing conditions and human processes in precise localities.

Ecological Interpretations

Ecological thinking applied to public health does not search for specific cause-effect relationships isolated from the contextual conditions in which people live. This kind of thinking recognizes the complexity and change stemming from either internal development or external influences, which can challenge both natural and built environments. Extreme weather events are one common example of this kind of challenge that can impact directly on health and well-being. Socio-ecological theories and concepts have been used increasingly since the 1980s to study environmental health in specific localities and especially in situations of change.[16]

Ecological interpretations of public health were proposed in the behavioral and social sciences that addressed people–environment relations as early as the 1950s.[17] For example, contributions in ecological psychology have applied the concepts of affordance, behavior setting and supportive environment to analyze specific kinds of human activities in precise types of settings including schools and public parks.[18] The World Health Organization "Strategy for Diet, Physical Activity and Obesity" is one example of the application of ecological interpretations in public health campaigns.[19] This approach has explicit implications for the design and layout of buildings, neighborhoods, cities and their hinterlands.

Ecological interpretations can provide a more comprehensive understanding of the multiple and mutual influence of variables on human health across a wide range of geographical spectrums from specific buildings and public spaces to neighborhoods and cities. In contrast to other interpretations of environmental health, ecological ones consider simultaneously the environmental and policy contexts of human life, as well as the cultural and social influences and specific psychological characteristics of humans.[20] Ecological interpretations explicitly account for multiple levels of influence, thus enabling the development of more comprehensive public health policies for coordinated interventions. They have been used to develop interventions that target change in environmental conditions (such as access to healthy food, or public green spaces) and specific human behavior at the personal, interpersonal and community levels (such as the promotion of active living to counteractive sedentary lifestyles).[21]

Behavioral interpretations consider only individual characteristics and nearby social influences while not accounting for the larger environmental conditions, community organization, economic development and public policies that influence human behavior and health. In contrast, ecological interpretations posit that a combination of individual, environment, societal and policy influences should be considered using an integrative approach. For example, the common request to provide green public spaces in urban areas is no assurance that people will use them to promote their health.

The main advantage of ecological interpretations is their focus on multiple levels of influence and the combined effect of different influences across a range of geographical scales. In particular, public policies intended to encourage designs of buildings and public spaces that promote health and well-being can impact entire populations, whereas those interventions that only target individuals may only achieve desired outcomes for those who choose to participate.

Principles of Healthy Residential Environments

Residential environments are known to influence quality of life and well-being following the results of numerous studies in a range of disciplines cited in the chapters in this book. The multiple components of housing units and outdoor areas, as reviewed in Table 2.1, need to be considered in terms of their potential and effective contribution to physical, social and mental health and well-being. In principle, there are eight main components that ought to be considered including:

1. The characteristics of the site, in ensuring safety from disasters including earthquakes, landslides, flooding and fires; and protection from any potential source of natural radon.[22]
2. The residential building as a shelter for inhabitants from the extremes of outdoor temperature; as a protector against dust, insects and rodents; as a provider of security from unwanted persons; and as an insulator against noise.[23,24]
3. The effective provision of a safe and continuous supply of water that meets standards for human consumption, and the maintenance of sewage and solid waste disposal.[25]
4. Ambient atmospheric conditions in the residential neighborhood and indoor air quality related to emissions from industrial production, transportation, fuels

used for domestic cooking and heating and the local climate and ventilation within and around buildings.[26]

5. Household occupancy conditions, which can influence the transmission of airborne infections including pneumonia and tuberculosis, and the incidence of injury from domestic accidents.[27]

6. Accessibility to community facilities and services (for commerce, education, employment, leisure and primary health care) which are affordable and available to all individuals and groups.[28]

7. Food safety, including to provision of uncontaminated fresh foods that can be stored with protection against spoilage.[29]

8. The control of vectors and hosts of disease outdoors and inside residential buildings which can propagate in the building structure; the use of non-toxic materials and finishes for housing and building construction; the use and storage of dangerous substances or equipment in the residential environment.[30,31]

Research in diverse disciplines since the 1990s confirms that the relations between residential environments and health are not limited to the above eight sets of criteria. The housing environment can also be considered in terms of its capacity to nurture and sustain social and psychological processes.[32] The multiple dimensions of residential environments that circumscribe the resident's capacity to use her/his domestic setting for restorative processes is included in a broad concept known as "the residential context of health."[33]

Other contributions confirm that achieving environmental quality across diverse geographical scales will depend as much on decisions about the use of resources including land, materials and methods to construct residential environments, as on the layout and volume of services and energy sources used to secure environmental conditions in buildings and urban neighborhoods.[34] The interrelations between indoor and outdoor environments are omnipresent. However, too frequently they are taken for granted. They are partly regulated by the activities and lifestyles of households. In several countries including New Zealand, for example, energy used in the building sector accounts for about half of all energy consumption, and buildings contribute to the "greenhouse effect" because they emit carbon dioxide along with other pollutants.[35] Studies in some industrialized countries show that more than half of all non-sleep activities of employed people between 18 and 64 years of age occur inside housing units. Children, the aged and housewives spend even more time indoors.[36] Consequently, any shortcomings in the indoor residential environment (including high household population density) may have implications on human health and well-being.[37]

If housing and the built environment are considered too narrowly, then the interrelations between housing, health and well-being may not seem important. An ecological perspective can provide a broad framework for comprehending the multiple dimensions of housing and health shown in Table 2.1 that ought to be identified and studied. This requires a shift from disciplinary sector-based contributions to intersectoral collaboration.

Intersectoral and Transdisciplinary Contributions

Our capacity to deal with complex subjects including how the housing in which we live can promote or harm health and well-being is insufficient for several reasons, including the diversity and complexity of this subject; the difficulty of identifying and measuring the interrelations between all the components of residential environments and health; and the need to understand the relative importance of these components in precise localities, and over time.[38] Therefore, it is suggested that it is necessary to shift from disciplinary and multi-disciplinary approaches to interdisciplinary and transdisciplinary contributions.

In this chapter, disciplinarity refers to the specialization and fragmentation of academic disciplines since the nineteenth century. Each discipline has its own concepts, definitions and methodological protocols for the study of its precisely defined domain of competence.[39] For example, in the domain of environmental sciences, different definitions, concepts and methods of what constitutes the environment coexist in biology, chemistry, geology and physics. This means that collaboration across disciplinary boundaries will not be easy until a common understanding is achieved.

Multi-disciplinary refers to an additive research agenda that accepts each researcher remaining within his/her discipline and applying its concepts and methods without collaboration with other researchers. This approach is still common in the environmental sciences and is frequently applied in environmental impact assessments of large-scale housing and urban development projects (EIA).

Interdisciplinary contributions involve concerted actions and integration that are applied by researchers in at least two different disciplines to achieve a shared goal about a common subject.[40] In contrast, transdisciplinary contributions incorporate a combination of concepts and knowledge used by academics, other researchers and actors in society, including representatives of the private sector, public administrations and citizens. These contributions enable the cross-fertilization of knowledge and experiences from diverse groups of people to promote an enlarged vision of a subject by concerted action that addresses real world situations.[41] Collaborative planning and participatory design are tangible ways of co-producing residential environments with the involvement of future residents.

Multidisciplinarity, interdisciplinarity and transdisciplinarity are complementary rather than being mutually exclusive. Both interdisciplinary and transdisciplinary research and practice require a common conceptual framework and analytical methods based on shared terminology, mental images and common goals. These need to be applied to co-create a shared vision of future residential neighborhoods and cities. There are numerous examples of project implementation, especially pragmatic responses to situations that involve a number of non-academic actors and institutions. These contributions challenge the long-standing divide between research and practice by implementing joint problem solving methods. During the definition and organization of transdisciplinary research programs and projects, the themes, subjects and research questions are not only selected with respect to perceived knowledge gaps identified by researchers but also by the priorities of representatives of specific groups (e.g. funding agencies, community associations, private enterprises, public administrations). This means that dialogue and negotiation processes are crucial to ensure the credibility, legitimacy and salience of selected subjects and research questions. In this respect, transdisciplinary contributions are quite different from basic research, interdisciplinary research and applied research.[42]

The World Health Organization Healthy Cities Project

The Healthy Cities project was founded in 1987 by 11 European cities and the WHO Regional Office for Europe. Today there are more than 30 national and regional networks in Europe involving about 600 municipalities, now complemented by many hundreds more in each of the regions of the world.[43] The Health for All Strategy provides the strategic framework for this project. The Healthy Cities project in the WHO European region includes four main components. First, the designated cities are committed to a comprehensive approach to achieving the goals of the project. Second, national and sub-national networks work together with EURONET in order to facilitate co-operation between partners. Third, multi-city action plans (MCAPs) are planned and implemented by networks of cities collaborating on specific issues of common interest. Finally, model projects are being implemented in central and eastern Europe.

The Healthy Cities project involves collaboration between sectors to define a "City Health Plan" that identifies the interrelations between living conditions in urban areas and the health of residents. Innovative projects show that health can be improved by addressing the physical environment, and the social and economic determinants of health in all situations (such as the home, the school, the workplace). This broad interpretation means that equity and social inequalities are identified as key factors in cities that need to be addressed. In particular, the plight of vulnerable social groups (including the handicapped, homeless, unemployed, single parents and street children) are ranked high for interventions. This approach is meant to focus on specific groups and particular neighborhoods where there are concentrations of vulnerable people with health risks.

European Policy Development on Housing and Health

Housing and health was attributed a high priority in 2004 at the Fourth European Ministerial Conference on Environment and Health. This decision by the Ministers of Environment and Health from more than 50 European countries reflected a growing concern about the health status of residents, especially those in urban areas.[44,45] The reasons for this concern are supported by information and data about rapid urbanization, increasing environmental, social and economic problems, and the health and well-being of specific social groups.

Design Implications

Architects, interior designers and housing authorities should accept that our habitat and housing conditions have a unique capacity to nurture and sustain biophysical and neuropsychological health, and other dimensions for a quality of life. For example, the possibility of a resident in her/his home environment to alleviate stress accumulated at school or in the workplace, and whether this capacity is mediated by views of nature or regular contact with natural surroundings such as urban parks. The multiple dimensions of housing that circumscribe the resident's capacity to use her/his domestic setting to promote well-being and quality of life is a subject that has been documented in academic and professional journals since the mid-nineteenth century. Today designers face the challenge to create housing conditions that can promote health for all kinds of households by reducing the risk of accidents, stress and enabling well-being. These dimensions of housing environments and the health of residents should not be isolated from diet, lifestyle, employment and the availability of affordable health care. A matrix of these dimensions, shown in Table 2.1, defines the multiple relations between housing and health across several different geo-political levels.

The ultimate goal of designing for health promotion is to combine research-based knowledge with professional know-how of practice. Knowledge for architects and urban designers has been accumulated by housing studies and epidemiological research but much of this evidence is still not used in practice today.[46] Overcoming this applicability gap is an important challenge for all those who wish to design for the promotion of health and quality of life.

Conclusion

At the beginning of the twenty-first century, it is necessary to reconsider health and housing in a broad environmental, economic, social and political context. Theoretical and methodological developments are necessary to formulate and apply a more comprehensive approach. Improved coordination of studies of the interrelations between housing, local environmental conditions and health is necessary.

If the ultimate goal of empirical studies is to influence policy decision-making in a number of sectors, including public health, housing and urban development, then there is an urgent need to promote multi-dimensional interpretations of health and illness. Today there is an urgent need for a new research agenda that addresses the following key issues:

1. Evidence from statistics and field studies that show a narrow focus on the individual cannot effectively address the social and economic factors that influence health. Area-based studies are necessary if the health of people in residential environments is to be dealt with in terms of context dependent inequalities and equity.
2. Precise mechanisms by which specific components of complicated residential environments influence health. Today, scientific knowledge and analytical

methods are not sufficiently developed to understand the combined effects of different types of risk factors in precise localities, for specific population groups and across different periods of exposure.

3. Conceptual clarification achieved by interdisciplinary collaboration. Health scientists, epidemiologists and family doctors can learn from housing researchers, architects and urban planners.

Evidence about how the socio-economic inequalities of people living in underprivileged housing areas impact on their health and well-being has increased since the 1990s.[47] Nonetheless, too little attention has been given to evaluating the effectiveness of interventions to promote health and well-being in specific localities and monitor the health outcomes. More research is required to evaluate different kinds of interventions that improve housing conditions and identify impacts on health and well-being by the collection of time series data. Environmental impact assessment (EIA), health impact assessment (HIA) and cost-benefit analysis (CBA) can be used to study interventions that are meant to promote health. These kinds of systematic evaluations could show that investments to improve housing and environmental quality extend beyond improving the built environment to promoting healthy lifestyles and reducing expenditure on treating illness and disease.

This chapter has shown that environmental, economic and social factors that influence health have locality specific characteristics and a temporal dimension, which need to be considered in terms of their combined effects as hazards to health and well-being. It has also shown that transdisciplinary interpretations of health and housing are necessary. Beyond disciplinary knowledge and expertise, transdisciplinary contributions are fruitful for addressing complex subjects like housing and health. Their future applications are an important challenge for the co-production of our future habitat.

Notes

1 Anthony McMichael, *Human Frontiers, Environments and Disease: Past Patterns, Uncertain Futures* (Cambridge: Cambridge University Press, 2001).
2 Michael Marmot, "Social Determinants of Health Inequalities," *Lancet* 365 (2005): 1099–1104.
3 Geof Rayner and Tim Lang, *Ecological Public Health: Reshaping the Conditions of Good Health* (Abington, UK, New York: Routledge, 2012).
4 James Sallis, Robert Cervero, William Ascher, Karla Henderson, M. Katherine Kraft, and Jacqueline Kerr, "An Ecological Approach to Creating Active Living Communities," *Annual Review of Public Health* 27 (2006): 297–322.
5 Roderick Lawrence, "Deciphering Interdisciplinary and Transdisciplinary Contributions," *Journal of Engineering and Science* 1 (2010): 125–130.
6 World Health Organization, *Constitution* (Geneva: World Health Organization, 1946).
7 Roderick Lawrence, "Housing and Health: From Interdisciplinary Principles to Transdisciplinary Research and Practice," *Futures* 36 (2004): 487–502.
8 Sallis, Cervero, Ascher, Henderson, Kraft, and Kerr, "An Ecological Approach."
9 Roderick Lawrence, "Building Healthy Cities: The World Health Organization Perspective," in *Handbook of Urban Health: Populations, Methods, and Practice*, eds. Sandro Galeo and David Vlahov (New York: Springer, 2005), 479–501.

10 Jan Golembiewski, "Moving From Theory to Praxis on the Fly; Introducing a Saluto-genic Method to Expedite Mental Healthcare Provision," *The Australian Journal of Emergency Management* 27 (2012): 42–47.

11 Rachel Dodge, Annette Daly, Jan Huyton, and Lalage Sanders, "The Challenge of Defining Well-Being," *International Journal of Well-being* 2 (2012): 222–235, doi:10.5502/ijw. v2i3.4.

12 Roderick Lawrence and Gilles Barbey, *Repenser l'habitat: donner un sens au logement* (Rethinking Habitats: Making Sense of Housing) (Paris; Golion: Infolio Editions, 2014).

13 Roderick Lawrence, "Human Ecology," in *Our Fragile World: Challenges and Opportunities for Sustainable Development*, Volume 1, ed. Mostafa K. Tolba (Oxford: EOLSS Publishers, 2001), 675–693.

14 Robert Dyball and Barry Newell, *Understanding Human Ecology: A Systems Approach to Sustainability* (Abington, UK; New York: Routledge, 2015).

15 John Turner, *Housing by People: Towards Autonomy in Building Environment* (New York: Pantheon Books, 1976).

16 Daniel Stokols, Shalini Misra, Miryha Gould Runnerstrom, and J. Aaron Hipp, "Psychology in an Age of Ecological Crisis: From Personal Angst to Collective Action," *American Psychologist* 64 (2009): 181–193.

17 Lawrence, "Human Ecology," 675–693.

18 Sallis, Cervero, Ascher, Henderson, Kraft, and Kerr, "An Ecological Approach," 297–322.

19 World Health Organization, *Strategy for Diet, Physical Activity and Obesity* (Geneva: World Health Organization, 2004).

20 Rayner and Lang, *Ecological Public Health*.

21 Hilary Thompson, Mark Petticrew, and David Morrison, "Health Effects of Housing Improvement: Systematic Review of Intervention Studies," *British Medical Journal* 323 (2001): 187–190.

22 Doocy Shannon, Amy Daniels, Sarah Murray, and Thomas Kirsch, "The Human Impact of Floods: A Historical Review of Events 1980–2009 and Systematic Literature Review," *PLoS Currents Disasters* (April 16, 2013), Edition 1, doi: 10.1371/currents.dis.f4deb4579 04936b07c09daa98ee8171a.

23 Matthias Braubach, David Jacobs, and David Ormandy, eds. *Environmental Burden of Disease Associated With Inadequate Housing: A Method Guide to the Quantification of Health Effects of Selected Housing Risks in the WHO European Region World Health Organization* (Copenhagen: World Health Organization, 2011).

24 James Krieger and Donna L. Higgins, "Housing and Health: Time Again for Public Health Action," *American Journal of Public Health* 92 (2002): 758–768.

25 United Nations, UN-Habitat, *Hidden Cities: Unmasking and Overcoming Inequalities in Health in Urban Areas*, UN-Habitat/WHO Report (Geneva: World Health Organization, 2010).

26 World Health Organization, Regional Office for Europe, *WHO Guidelines for Indoor Air Quality: Dampness and Mould* (Copenhagen: World Health Organization, 2009).

27 Claudia Solari and Robert Mare, "Housing Crowding Effects on Children's Wellbeing," *Social Science Research* 41 (2012): 464–476.

28 Galea Sandro and David Vlahov, eds. *Handbook of Urban Health: Populations, Methods and Practice* (New York: Springer, 2005).

29 Elizabeth Scott, "Food Safety and Foodborne Disease in 21st Century Homes," *The Canadian Journal of Infectious Diseases* 14 (2003): 277–280.

30 Krieger and Higgins, "Housing and Health," 758–768.

31 Tunga Salthammer, Sibel Mentese, and Rainer Marutzky, "Formaldehyde in the Indoor Environment," *Chemical Reviews* 110 (2010): 2536–2572.

32 Grace Campagna, "Linking Crowding, Housing Inadequacy, and Perceived Housing Stress," *Journal of Environmental Psychology* 45 (2016): 252–266.

33 Terry Hartig and Roderick Lawrence, eds. "The Residential Context of Health," *Journal of Social Issues* 59 (2003): 455–650 (special issue).

34 United Nations, UN-Habitat, *Hidden Cities: Unmasking and Overcoming Inequalities in Health in Urban Areas* (Geneva: World Health Organization, 2010).

35 Philippa Howden-Chapman and Ralph Chapman, "Health Co-Benefits From Housing-Related Policies," *Current Opinion in Environmental Sustainability* 4 (2012): 414–419.

36 Michael Baker, Michael Keall, Ee Lyn Au, and Philippa Howden-Chapman, "Home Is Where the Heart Is—Most of the Time," *New Zealand Medical Journal* 120 (2007): 1264.

37 David Ormandy, ed. *Housing and Health in Europe: The WHO LARES Project* (London; New York: Routledge, 2009).

38 Lawrence, "Housing and Health," 487–502.

39 Lawrence, "Deciphering Interdisciplinary," 125–130.

40 Roderick Lawrence, "Beyond Disciplinary Confinement to Imaginative Transdisciplinarity," in *Tackling Wicked Problems Through Transdisciplinary Imagination*, eds. Valerie Brown, John Harris, and Jacqueline Russell (London, UK: Earthscan, 2010), 16–30.

41 Roderick Lawrence, "Advances in Transdisciplinarity: Epistemologies, Methodologies and Processes," *Futures* 65 (2015): 1–9.

42 Gertrude Hirsch Hadorn, Holger Hoffmann-Riem, Susette Biber-Klemm, Walter Grossenbacher-Mansuy, Dominique Joye, Christian Pohl, Urs Wiesmann, and Elisabeth Zemp, eds. *Handbook of Transdisciplinary Research* (Berlin, Germany: Springer, 2008).

43 Lawrence, "Building Healthy Cities," 479–501.

44 WHO Regional Office for Europe, *Large Analysis and Review of European Housing and Health Status* (LARES) (Copenhagen: World Health Organization, 2007).

45 Xavier Bonneyfoy, Matthais Braubach, Maggie Davidson, and Nathalie Robbel, "A Pan-European Housing and Health Survey: Description and Evaluation of Methods and Approaches," *International Journal of Environment and Pollution* 30 (2007): 363–383.

46 Roderick Lawrence, "Mind the Gap: Bridging the Divide Between Knowledge, Policy and Practice," in *The Routledge Handbook of Planning for Health and Well-Being*, eds. Hugh Barton, Susan Thompson, Sarah Burgess, and Marcus Grant (New York; London UK: Routledge, 2015), 74–84.

47 Thompson, Petticrew, and Morrison, "Health Effects of Housing Improvement," 187–190.

Sites

World Health Organization Large Analysis and Review of European Housing and Health Status
www.euro.who.int/Housing/lares/20080403_1
World Health Organization Healthy Cities Project
www.euro.who.int/en/health-topics/environment-and-health/urban-health/activities/healthy-cities

3

HUMAN FACTORS AND ERGONOMICS THROUGH THE LIFESPAN

Sue Hignett, Sharon Cook, Martin Maguire, and Ellen Taylor

Introduction

Designers of today's environments face unprecedented challenges in accommodating an increasingly diverse population across characteristics including age, disability, ethnicity, gender alignment and religion; Eliciting, and working to meet the associated population needs is achieved through the application of a Human Factors and Ergonomics (HFE) approach. This chapter will inform designers of the role of HFE within interior architecture with specific consideration of design challenges across the lifespan in promoting health and well-being. It will demonstrate how design can meet physical, sensory, cognitive and emotional needs over a variety of environments including: workplaces, schools, domestic settings, care homes, hospitals and transport.

Human Factors and Ergonomics in Architecture

There has been a tendency to use the term 'Ergonomics' to refer to interactions with the physical environment, and 'Human Factors' in connection with psychological and organizational issues. However, from both theoretical and professional perspectives, one cannot be considered without the other, so the terms are now used interchangeably.[1,2] Given the wide range of interactions which people undertake within interior architecture, it is evident that each term in its own right is applicable in this context and so the term HFE will be used within this chapter.

The role of HFE is to apply a scientific approach to the design of the systems (micro and macro) in which people interact with their physical, organizational and social environments to give the two key outcomes of optimizing human well-being and performance.[3] Fundamental to this optimization is the need to ensure that the design of the environment and the activities within it support the needs of the users.

Defining the Environment in HFE

From an HFE perspective, the human–physical environment interface[4] often over-laps with HFE domains of cognition and organization. However, the focus is often air quality, noise, illumination and vibration, or more locally, workstations, indi-vidual products, or equipment and furnishings, rather than the larger-scale concepts associated with spatial layouts or with other aspects of the system.[5,6,7,8] As a result of this lack of clarity, four subset 'components' of the HFE environment have been drawn from the literature:[9]

1) Workspace Envelope: the wider workplace including the building characteris-tics, arrangement of personal workspace components and space constraints.
2) Personal Workspace: the layout of the "workstation" or immediate area of use, including the relationship of equipment, furniture and controls available to the user (including anthropometry).
3) Products: the selection/specification of equipment, furniture or controls.
4) Ambient Environment: the physical environment of thermal, air, noise, visual and illumination considerations.

When to Consider HFE in Design of the Environment

When developing the built environment, there is acceptance that problems addressed early in design require reduced effort and expense to fix than those later in design, production or use,[10,11] and this can be especially important in the context of safety considerations.[12] Within the Safety Risk Assessment Toolkit for the Design of Healthcare Settings, a cost-influence curve was developed to illustrate the impact of moving safety upstream in the design process.[13] The curve differentiates between the ability to influence the life cycle costs of a building project through a proactive design approach as compared to a more costly process of retrofitting. Changes early in design are less expensive but increase in cost through construction and occu-pancy; the highest costs relate to the long-term impact of recurrent adverse events over the life cycle of a building, often 30–50 years or more. Likewise, HFE efforts are better placed early in design.

Applying HFE Principles in Design

Hignett[14] argues that poor design can permeate throughout the system requir-ing reliance on human adaptation (coping) rather than beginning with a design that does not require behavior change. This is fitting the user to the environment, rather than fitting the environment to the user.[15,16] To understand fit, however, it is important to understand the active participants and general conditions of human performance, behavior and user characteristics. For example, in considering safety in health care design, safety is a result of the complexity of the organization, peo-ple and environment (SCOPE).[17] Designing with HFE principles establishes a

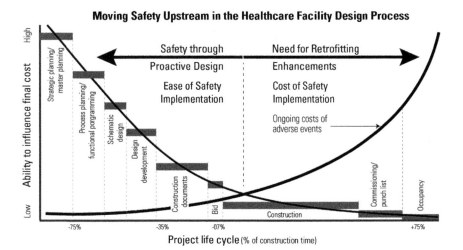

FIGURE 3.1   The Cost-Influence Curve in Design

Source: Adapted from Taylor, Hignett, and Joseph, 2014

TABLE 3.1   Designing for Falls with DEEP SCOPE

		Decision-making	*Movement*	*Perception*	*Strength*	*Manipulation*
Organization (Operations/ Policy)		Considera-tion 1				
People	Patients	Considera-tion 2				
	Staff	Considera-tion 3		Consider-ation 4		
Environment (Building Design)	Workspace envelope					
	Personal workspace Products	Considera-tion 5				
	Ambient environment	Considera-tion 6				

Source: Adapted from Taylor, 2016

framework to investigate complex systems relationships of the organization, people and environment for particular outcomes such as falls (see Figure 3.1).[18] This can be represented as a matrix of design considerations, as shown in Table 3.1.

HFE Methods

A variety of methods for identifying, measuring and evaluating user requirements can be applied to ensure that key issues have been identified and resolved. It is important that user needs remain at the forefront of this iterative process with both direct user involvement and indirect representation via user data and models. Typical HFE methods include:

1) *Anthropometry:* human body measurements of size, shape, strength, mobility, flexibility and working capacity.[19] This branch of HFE provides data to match the physical demands of the environment with human limitations and capabilities.

2) *Hierarchical Task Analysis (HTA):* describes a task as a higher level goal (e.g., safe transportation of medicine) with a hierarchy of subordinate task steps. At each level of the subtasks a plan is used to direct (inform) the sequence and possible variance of task steps.[20] It has been used to describe system dynamics and human-system interfaces.[21]

3) *Interviews and surveys:* to obtain first-hand accounts from people about their activities and tasks during daily life.[22] This includes knowledge elicitation from domain experts[23] as well as participant (user) involvement in HCD.[24]

4) *Link analysis:* uses observations to collect data about the interactions between components in a system (task activities and physical/cognitive relationships) to provide outputs as spatial diagrams.[25]

5) *Empathic modeling:* where designers engage with a simulation device to help understand the user's perspective in the outside world, e.g., to use a wheelchair for a day.[26] This method has been used in architectural projects and is taught in architectural programs within HFE modules.[27]

6) *User trials:* are often used with detailed scenarios (based on task analysis) within a simulated environment (mock-up) to allow a systematic evaluation of the design under controlled conditions.[28]

7) *Design Decision Groups:* a participatory HFE approach which combines several methods including word map, round-robin questionnaires, layout modeling, silent drawing and mock-ups. This systematic approach is used for workplace layout and design to create shared experience events.[29]

HFE Examples across the Lifespan

A number of case studies across the life span are presented to demonstrate the embodiment of the HFE approach in the design of interior architecture for health and well-being. A range of human characteristics are addressed, HFE methods illustrated and domain applications showcased.

Early Life

Case Study 1: Improving the Birthing Experience

The benefits/risks associated with water birth have been discussed by the medical profession and by patients (mothers) and it is suggested that the 'enveloping effect of the water wrapped the women in warmth and provided a sense of privacy, whilst enabling them to deal with their pain without the need for pharmacological pain relief.'[30] However, the design of birthing pools (large barrels) created a barrier for use with mothers finding it very difficult to get into the birthing pool and almost impossible to get out in an emergency. As part of an HFE project, a detailed analysis was carried out to map the stakeholders:

1) Mothers (and their partners): enter/exit the pool; support in a range of positions during labor.
2) Clinical staff: care for the mother including examinations and monitoring.
3) Baby: may need emergency assistance.
4) Maintenance, cleaning and infection control support staff.

An iterative prototyping approach was taken, including a scale mock-up which was evaluated in the hospital. A new birthing pool was designed to support independent access/egress with steps and hand rails; a range of labor and birthing positions; staff examinations using a concave side; and delivery and perineal examination plus emergency exit of the mother via a horse-shoe shaped seat. This HFE design project revolutionized the design of birthing pools resulting in its international adoption.[31]

Case Study 2: Design for Neonatal Intensive Care Unit (NICU)

In the United Kingdom (UK), the NICU is often one large, open room with the cots (incubators) side by side. This has observation and access advantages but disadvantages relating to noise, lighting and privacy.[32,33] Recently, there has been increased provision of single rooms aiming to improve privacy and reduce movement (and infection transmission risks) around the unit and between departments.[34,35] The Department of Health[36] responded to these changes in clinical care by conducting a review of UK design guidelines for neonatal units to determine the space required to care for and treat neonates. They engaged an HFE team to look at the spatial requirements using a 5-step process[37] to support decision-making for clinical space planning in health care facilities by:

1) Defining the clinical specialty and space.
2) Collecting data (using task analysis methods) with clinical staff and neonates to produce a simulation scenario representing the frequent and safety-critical activities.
3) Calculating the average spatial requirements through functional space experiments.
4) Incorporating additional data for storage and circulation to produce a spatial recommendation.
5) Reviewing and verifying the recommendations to consider alternative layouts and technology.

HTA and LA were used to understand and evaluate space use and then develop a test scenario on the basis of the frequency and criticality of activities.[38,39] Clinical tasks were observed with 28 staff providing care to 15 newborn babies and staff actions/task behaviors were recorded for 21 clinicians using multi-directional video data to plot the movements of each participant, equipment and furniture during the tasks.

It was found that there was no family space for the parents to stay with their child; storage was limited; there were no nursing trolleys and clinical bins in the cot space; and staff sometimes worked in awkward positions due to the cramped space. Recommendations were made for the dimensions of individual clinical neonatal cot space (13.50 m² [or 145.3 ft²], width 4.13 m [or 13.6 ft] × length 3.27 m [or 10.7 ft]); these were reviewed and validated by the expert group.[40] The complexity of the spatial requirements suggests that circulation and storage considerations must be included for both single and multiple NICU cot spaces.

Child to Adult

Case Study 3: School Design

The design of the educational environment has many HFE challenges in relation to furniture, classroom layout, equipment, individual storage, lighting and ventilation. A useful overview of design issues for school stakeholders is offered by Nair and Fielding[41] in the context of both construction and renovation of schools, and evaluation of the educational adequacy of existing school facilities.

Both neck and back pain have been researched with significant association reported for school furniture features, school bag weight as well as family history and personal problems (emotional and conduct).[42] Milanese and Grimmer[43] investigated the relationship between reported back problems in an adolescent student population and the match between their individual anthropometric dimensions and their school furniture. Data was collected from 1269 pupils to investigate back pain symptoms and anthropometric challenges. Overall, a higher probability of reporting back pain was found for students with anthropometric dimensions in the fourth quartile (the tallest students). Detailed anthropometric measurements were collected to investigate furniture incompatibility for 180 children (7–12 years) in Greece for stature, elbow height, shoulder height, upper arm length, knee height, popliteal height and buttock-popliteal length. It was found that chairs were too high and too deep and desks were too high.[44] School furniture that is too low or too small can also be a problem. There are now design standards for school furniture to prevent the exposure to these musculoskeletal risks.[45]

Case Study 4: Design for Adolescents

Adolescence covers the life period of 10 to 19 years[46] when individuals grow from dependent children into independent adults. Lang et al.[47] explored the different design requirements that might improve compliance with medical device use during this changing period. They found that usability could be improved by allowing a level of customization (both for operation and appearance).

One difference in the use of the built environment has been identified for younger wheelchair users when designing their workspace where it cannot be assumed that an individual will transfer from their wheelchair to local seating. Nowak reported that adolescents preferred to stay in their wheelchair to avoid both additional effort and asking for assistance.[48] For interior architecture this has two ramifications in providing interfaces (built and furniture) suitable for wheelchairs but also providing space to include the wheelchair as an additional piece of furniture (with storage/space for rejected seating).

There is limited research on this age group, but the included studies point to the development of individual preferences as more choice becomes available with increasing independence.

Growing Older

Case Study 5: Workstation Design

This case study focuses on the personal workspace associated with computer use, a pertinent concern given their widespread use for work or leisure. A workstation assessment considers the extent to which the task and environment contribute to the users' health and well-being with the aim of promoting safe, comfortable and efficient engagement with associated activities. By assessing people's abilities and limitations, their jobs, equipment and working environment and the interaction between them, it is possible to design safe, effective and productive work systems.[49] Ergonomics advice is available, often in the form of generic guidelines such the Computer workstations e-Tool[50] and Display Screen Equipment (DSE) workstation checklist[51] and personalized health solutions can be developed as the following case study illustrates.

An office worker experienced cold extremities due to Raynaud's Syndrome, musculoskeletal pains and visual discomfort. The design of the workstation and work flow was investigated through measurement of the workplace, observation of working practices and application of relevant regulations. Physical and procedural adjustments were recommended including a heated footrest to reduce the Raynaud's Syndrome symptoms, document holder and re-location of the hard drive (to reduce the musculoskeletal strain), second screen to reduce visual discomfort, and advice on the need for breaks and postural change. This HFE approach resulted in low-cost solutions which reduced discomfort, improved morale and reduced the risk of absenteeism.[52]

Case Study 6: Empathic Modeling

As the global population ages, designers can often be younger than those for whom they are designing. It has been suggested that there is a need to increase awareness and understanding of users with different capabilities, limitations and needs—also known as stretching the Empathic Horizon.[53] Human–Centered Design (HCD) as a component of a wider HFE approach, for example, investigating 'why, how and what'[54] as part of a wider HFE approach which will also include 'who, where and when.'[55] The HCD cycle is an established model to incorporate user needs and desires based on the international standard ISO 9241–210.[56]

This can be facilitated through the use of empathic-modeling tools, such as LUSKInS (Loughborough University Sensory and Kinesthetic Interactive Simulations). This range of wearable simulations supports designers in their understanding of the health conditions of others by enabling direct experience of some of the associated symptoms and their consequent impacts to daily living.[57]

Drawing on primary and secondary data, the first LUSKInS (Third Age Suit), a whole-body wearable simulation, was developed for the Ford Motor Company to simulate aspects of reduced joint mobility, tactile sensitivity and vision.[58] The simulation was then transferred to the aerospace industry via a technology-sharing alliance, leading to an improvement in the design of the aircraft environment in terms of visibility and physical access. It has subsequently been used by architects as part of a hospital design program, where the architects 'found the simplest of tasks, such as sitting down, standing up and reaching out the arm became laboured and difficult when wearing the suit.'[59] The psychological impact of reduced confidence due to the increased challenges when interacting with the environment were reported,[60] which emphasizes the importance of considering all aspects of human-environment interactions.

Case Study 7: Kitchen Design

The Instrumental Activities of Daily Living (IADLs) define daily activities supporting independent living within the community and include meal preparation, which has implications for the role of kitchen design.[61] A research program project 'Transitions in Kitchen Living' investigated the problems and needs of older people when using their kitchens independently.[62] Interviews with 48 older people who lived in a variety of homes including detached houses, apartments and sheltered accommodation, identified a number of issues including:

1) Wall cupboard shelves too high.
2) Poor lighting, especially in the cooking area.
3) Window handles difficult to reach.
4) Sinks and worktops at an inconvenient height.
5) No space for a table for seated activity.

Coping strategies had been developed including stools or steps, installing table lamps or stick-on LED lights. Other adaptations had been made at the installation stage, for example by fitting cupboards at more convenient heights.

Through a HFE approach, kitchen designs, which adapt to users' needs (as they age) could include pull-down wall cupboards, adjustable height work surfaces and the installation of mid-level ovens to eliminate the need for reaching and bending. The challenge is to make kitchen flexibility a market standard so that everyone can use their kitchen optimally.

Case Study 8: Design of Dementia Care Environments

Dementia is predicted to become increasingly prevalent in the future,[63] creating a challenge in providing appropriate housing where the design of the environment can contribute towards the management of illness.[64] As the demography of higher income countries changes and the baby boomer generation ages there are more older (and oldest old) being cared for in specialist facilities.[65] Care environments specifically designed for dementia can help maintain or foster a sense of independence, and encourage participation in activities which could potentially maintain a higher quality of life for longer.[66]

To explore this area further, a review of the guidelines for dementia design was undertaken which found inconsistencies in the advice.[67] A systematic literature review was then undertaken to investigate the robustness of the guidance in terms of degree of variance and whether HFE principles had been considered. An initial scoping study mapped key HFE issues relating to the design of dementia care environments to illustrate different dementia diagnoses, physical, emotional and psychological needs, design challenges and research (investigation) methods (see Figure 3.2).

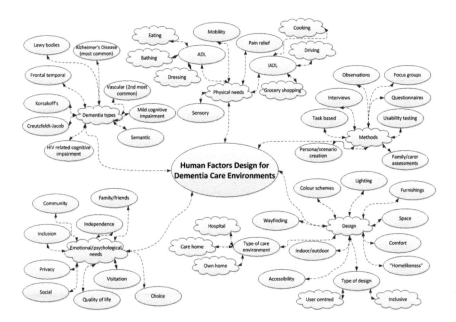

FIGURE 3.2   Design for Dementia Mind Map

Source: Jais et al., 2015

The complexity of the design challenge can be illustrated when a combination of negative environmental conditions such as lack of lighting, poor air quality (including odors from cleaning products),[68] excessive temperatures and high noise levels contributed to wandering and agitated behaviors.[69,70,71,72] Conversely, higher levels of lighting, lower levels of noise, good air quality and an ambient temperature were linked to improved nutritional intake[73] and being able to smell cooking was thought to boost nutritional intake as an appetite stimulant.[74]

Conclusion

Within this chapter the role of HFE expertise and methods have been outlined in the design of environments through the lifespan. An HFE approach can support the design of more accommodating (better fit and more useable) environments by ensuring that user needs are identified and met. In addition to improving performance (human–environment interactions) there may be cost-saving benefits through reduced accidents, improved well-being and living independently for longer. Including HFE knowledge and principle early in the design process will be less expensive with maximum benefits from including HFE expertise as part of the design team. The case studies demonstrate that HFE can make valuable contributions to health and well-being across the life course through the application of a range research and evaluation methods.

Notes

1 Sue Hignett, Pascale Carayon, Peter Buckle, and Ken Catchpole, "State of Science: Human Factors and Ergonomics in Healthcare," *Ergonomics* 56, no. 10 (2013): 1491–1503.
2 John R. Wilson and Sarah Sharples, *Evaluation of Human Work*, 4th edition (Boca Raton, FL: CRC Press, 2015).
3 Jan Dul, Ralph Bruder, Peter Buckle, Pascale Carayon, Pierre Falzon, William S. Marras, John R. Wilson, and Bas van der Doelen, "A Strategy for Human Factors/Ergonomics: Developing the Discipline and Profession," *Ergonomics* 55, no. 4 (2012): 377–395.
4 Pascale Carayon, *Handbook of Human Factors and Ergonomics in Health Care and Patient Safety*, 2nd edition (Boca Raton, FL: CRC Press, 2011).
5 Mark S. Sanders and Ernest J. McCormick, *Human Factors in Engineering and Design*, 7th edition (New York: McGraw-Hill Education, 1993).
6 Christopher D. Wickens, Justin G. Hollands, and Raja Parasuraman, *Engineering Psychology & Human Performance*, 4th edition (Boston, MA: Pearson Education, 2013).
7 Carayon, *Handbook of Human Factors and Ergonomics*.
8 Erminia Attaianese and Gabriella Duca, "Human Factors and Ergonomic Principles in Building Design for Life and Work Activities: An Applied Methodology," *Theoretical Issues in Ergonomics Science* 13, no. 2 (2012): 187–202.
9 Ellen Taylor and Sue Hignett, "The SCOPE of Hospital Falls: A Systematic Mixed Studies Review," *HERD: Health Environments Research & Design* 9 (2016): 86–109.
10 Max Wideman, "Managing the Development of Building Projects for Better Results," Webinar based on published 1981 paper presented at the AEW Services, AEW Services, Vancouver, BC, 1–14, http://maxwideman.com/papers/managing/MngPrjDev4Rslt.pdf.
11 Alan Griffith and Anthony Charles Sidwell, "Development of Constructability Concepts, Principles and Practices," *Construction and Architectural Management* 4, no. 4 (1997): 295–310.

12 Wayne C. Christensen, "Safety Through Design," *Professional Safety* 48, no. 3 (2003): 32–39.
13 Ellen Taylor, Sue Hignett, and Anjali Joseph, "The Environment of Safe Care: Considering Building Design as One Facet of Safety," in *Proceedings of the International Symposium on Human Factors and Ergonomics in Health Care* (Chicago: Sage publishing with the Human Factors and Ergonomics Society, 2014), 123–127.
14 Sue Hignett, "Why Design Starts With People," Patient Safety Resource Centre: The Health Foundation, 1–5, http://patientsafety.health.org.uk/sites/default/files/resources/why_design_starts_with_people.pdf.
15 Dul, Bruder, Buckle, Carayon, Falzon, Marras, Wilson, and van der Doelen. "A Strategy for Human Factors."
16 Ibid.
17 Taylor and Hignett, "The SCOPE of Hospital Falls."
18 Ellen Taylor, "Anticipate to Participate to Integrate: Bridging Evidence-Based Design and Human Factors Ergonomics to Advance Safer Healthcare Facility Design," *Ph.D. Thesis*, Design School, 2016.
19 Stephen Pheasant and Christine M. Haslegrave, *Anthropometry, Ergonomics and the Design of Work*, 3rd edition (Boca Raton, FL: Taylor & Francis, 2005).
20 Andrew Shepherd, *Hierarchical Task Analysis* (London, UK: Taylor & Francis, 2001).
21 Neville A. Stanton, "Hierarchical Task Analysis: Developments, Applications and Extensions," *Applied Ergonomics* 37 (2006): 55–79.
22 C. Robson, *Real World Research*, 3rd edition (Chichester, West Sussex: Wiley-Blackwell, 2011).
23 Nigel R. Shadbolt and Paul R. Smart, "Chapter 7, Knowledge Elicitation: Methods, Tools and Techniques," in *Evaluation of Human Work*, 4th edition, eds. John R. Wilson and Sarah Sharples (Boca Raton, FL: CRC Press, 2015), 163–200.
24 David Kirk, Ian McClelland, and Jane Fulton Sari, "Chapter 10, Involving People in Design Research," in *Evaluation of Human Work*, 4th edition, eds. John R. Wilson and Sarah Sharples (Boca Raton, FL: CRC Press, 2015), 249–298.
25 Neville A. Stanton and Mark S. Young, *A Guide to Methodology in Ergonomics* (London, UK: Taylor & Francis, 1999).
26 Colette Nicolle and Martin Maguire, "Empathic Modelling in Teaching Design for All," in *Proceedings of the Tenth International Conference on Human-Computer Interaction, Section: Universal Access in HCI—Inclusive Design in the Information Society*, Vol. 4, June 22–27, ed. C. Stephanidis (Greece, Lawrence Erlbaum Associates, Inc., 2003), 143–147.
27 Burcak Altay and Halime Demirkan, "Inclusive Design: Developing Students' Knowledge and Attitude Through Empathic Modelling," *International Journal of Inclusive Education* 18, no. 2 (2014): 196–217.
28 Kirk, McClelland, and Sari, "Chapter 10, Involving People in Design Research."
29 Diane Gyi, Sally Shalloe, and John R. Wilson, Chapter 34, "Participatory Ergonomics," in *Evaluation of Human Work*, 4th edition, eds. John R. Wilson and Sarah Sharples (Boca Raton, FL: CRC Press, 2015), 883–906.
30 Robyn M. Maude and Maralyn J. Foureur, "It's Beyond Water: Stories of Women's Experience of Using Water for Labour and Birth," *Women and Birth* 20 (2007): 17–24.
31 Matt Chorley, "£10 Million Fund for Hospitals to Buy More Birthing Pools and Chairs for New Mums," www.dailymail.co.uk/news/article-2535103/10million-maternity-fund-hospitals.html.
32 Robert D. White, "The Physical Environment of the Neonatal Intensive Care Unit—Implications for Premature Newborns and Their Care-Givers" [business briefing], *US Pediatr Care* (2005): 13–14.
33 Phyllis Brown and Lauren T. Taquino, "Designing and Delivering Neonatal Care in Single Rooms," *Journal of Perinatal and Neonatal Nursing* 15, no. 1 (2001): 68–83.
34 Robert D. White, "The 7th Consensus Committee on Recommended Design Standards for Advanced Neonatal Care," Recommended Standards for Newborn ICU Design, 2007, www3.nd.edu/~nicudes/Recommended%20Standards%207%20final%20may%2015.pdf.

35 Mardelle M. Shepley, Debra D. Harris, and Robert White, "Open Bay and Single Family Room Neonatal Intensive Care Units," *Environmental Behaviour* 40, no. 2 (2008): 249–268.

36 White, "Consensus Committee."

37 Sue Hignett, Jun Lu, and Kevin Morgan, "Empirical Review of NHS Estates Ergonomic Drawings," Department of Health Estates and Facilities Management Research Report No. B(02)13, The Stationary Office, London, UK, 2008.

38 Bryce G. Rutter, "Designing the Ergonomically Correct Medical Environment, Proceedings of the 8th Symposium on Healthcare Design; San Diego, California," *Journal of Healthcare Design* 8 (1996): 127–131.

39 Sue Hignett and Jun Lu, "An Investigation of the Use of Health Building Notes By UK Healthcare Building Designers," *Applied Ergonomics* 40 (2009): 608–616.

40 Sue Hignett, Jun Lu, and Mike Fray, "Observational Study of Treatment Space in Individual Neonatal Cot Spaces," *Journal of Perinatal and Neonatal Nursing* 24, no. 3 (2010): 267–273.

41 Prakash Nair and Randall Fielding, *The Language of School Design: Design Patterns for 21st Century Schools*, 3rd edition (2005), DesignShare.com.

42 Sam Murphy, Peter Buckle, and David Stubbs, "A Cross-Sectional Study of Self-Reported Back and Neck Pain Among English Schoolchildren and Associated Physical and Psychological Risk Factors," *Applied Ergonomics* 38, no. 6 (2007): 797–804.

43 Steve Milanese and Kevin Grimmer, "School Furniture and the User Population: An Anthropometric Perspective," *Ergonomics* 47, no. 4 (2004): 416–426.

44 Georgia Panagiotopoulou, Kosmas Christoulas, Anthoula Papanckolaou, and Konstantinos Mandroukas, "Classroom Furniture Dimensions and Anthropometric Measures in Primary School," *Applied Ergonomics* 35 (2004): 121–128.

45 BS EN 1729-1:2015, Furniture, Chairs and Tables for Educational Institutions, Functional Dimensions, http://shop.bsigroup.com/ProductDetail/?pid=000000000030263209.

46 WHO, *The Second Decade: Improving Adolescent Health and Development* (Geneva: World Health Organization, 2001).

47 Alexandra L. Lang, Jennifer L. Martin, Sarah Sharples, and John A. Crowe, "The Effect of Design on the Usability and Real World Effectiveness of Medical Devices: A Case Study With Adolescent Users," *Applied Ergonomics* 44 (2013): 799–810.

48 Ewa Nowak, "Workspace for Disabled People," *Ergonomics* 32 (1989): 9, 1077–1088.

49 Health and Safety Executive, *Ergonomics and Human Factors at Work—A Brief Guide*, www.hse.gov.uk/pubns/indg90.pdf.

50 Occupational Safety and Health Administration, *Computer workstations e-Tool*, United States Department of Labor, www.osha.gov/SLTC/etools/computerworkstations/index.html.

51 Health and Safety Executive, *Display Screen Equipment (DSE) Workstation Checklist*, www.hse.gov.uk/pubns/ck1.htm.

52 Chartered Institute of Ergonomics and Human Factors, *Improving a Computer User's Comfort*, www.ergonomics.org.uk/wp-content/uploads/2015/05/8-Improving-a-computer-users-comfort.pdf.

53 Merlijn Kouprie and Froukje Sleeswijk Visser, "A Framework for Empathy in Design: Stepping Into and Out of the User's Life," *Journal of Engineering Design* 20, no. 5 (2009): 437–448.

54 Joyce Thomas and Deana McDonagh, "Empathic Design: Research Strategies," *Australasian Medical Journal* 6, no. 1 (2013): 1–6.

55 S. Hignett, "Healthcare Ergonomics: Reaching Out Into All Areas of Clinical Practice or 'Touching and Analysing the Elephant,'" *Proceedings of the 19th Triennial Conference of the International Ergonomics Association*, Melbourne, Australia, August 11–15, 2015.

56 ISO 9241-210, Ergonomics of Human-System Interaction, 2010, www.iso.org/obp/ui/#iso:std:iso:9241:-210:ed-1:v1:en.

57 Sharon Cook, John Richardson, Alastair Gibb, and Phil Bust, "Raising Awareness of the Occupational Health of Older Construction Workers," *CIB WO99 International Conference*, Melbourne, Australia, 2009.

58 David Hitchcock, Suzanne Lockyer, Sharon Cook, and Claire Quigley, "Third Age Usability and Safety—An Ergonomics Contribution to Design," *International Journal of Human-Computer Studies* 55, no. 4 (2001): 635–643.

59 "The Suit That Makes You Feel Old," *BBC News*, http://news.bbc.co.uk/1/hi/health/3538220.stm.

60 K. Spicer, "What's Old Is New—Engineers, Designers Walk in the Shoes of Older Passengers to Understand Needs of Future Air Travellers," *Boeing Frontiers* 4 (2005): 8, www.boeing.com/news/frontiers/i_ca1.html.

61 David A. Cromwell, Kathy Eagar, and Roslyn G. Poulos, "The Performance of Instrumental Activities of Daily Living Scale in Screening for Cognitive Impairment in Elderly Community Residents," *Journal of Clinical Epidemiology* 56, no. 2 (2003): 131–137.

62 Martin Maguire, Sheila Peace, Colette Nicolle, Russell Marshall, Ruth Sims, John Percival, and Clare Lawton, "Kitchen Living in Later Life: Exploring Ergonomic Problems, Coping Strategies and Design Solutions," *International Journal of Design* 8, no. 1 (2014): 73–91.

63 Cleusa P. Ferri, Martin Prince, Carol Brayne, Henry Brodaty, Laura Fratiglioni, Mary Ganguli, Kathleen Hall, Kazuo Hasegawa, Hugh Hendrie, Yueqin Huang, Anthony Jorm, Colin Mathers, Paulo Menezes, Elizabeth Rimmer, Marcia Scazufca. "Global Prevalence of Dementia: a Delphi Consensus Study," *Lancet*, 366, no. 9503, (2005): 2112–2117.

64 Kristen Day, Daisy Carreon, and Cheryl Stump, "The Therapeutic Design of Environments for People With Dementia: A Review of the Empirical Research," *The Gerontologist* 40, no. 4 (2000): 397–416.

65 Joseph Kandel and Christine Adamec, *The Encyclopedia of Elder Care* (New York: Infobase Publishing, 2009).

66 Jennifer Boger, Tammy Craig, and Alex Mihailidis, "Examining the Impact of Familiarity on Faucet Usability for Older Adults With Dementia," *BMC Geriatrics* 13 (2013): 63–75.

67 Charlotte Jais, Sue Hignett, Martin Habell, and Eef Hogervorst, "How Can Human Factors Be Used in the Design of Dementia Care Environments?" *Proceedings of European Healthcare Design Conference*, (London, UK: Royal College of Physicians, 2015).

68 Jonas E. Andersson, "'Touching Up' Communal Space of a Residential Home Setting: A Comparative Study of Tools for Assessing Changes in the Interior Architectural Space," *Journal of Housing for the Elderly* 25, no. 2 (2011): 175–216.

69 Donna L. Algase, Elizabeth R. A. Beattie, Cathy Antonakos, Cynthia A. Beel-Bates, and Lan Yao, "Wandering and the Physical Environment," *American Journal of Alzheimer's Disease and Other Dementias* 25, no. 4 (2010): 340–346.

70 Josep Garre-Olmo, Secundino López-Pousa, Antoni Turon-Estrada, Dolors Juvinyà, David Ballester, and Joan Vilalta-Franch, "Environmental Determinants of Quality of Life in Nursing Home Residents With Severe Dementia," *Journal of the American Geriatrics Society* 60, no. 7 (2012): 1230–1236.

71 Johnny K. W. Wong, Martin Skitmore, L. Laurie Buys, and Kai Wang, "The Effects of the Indoor Environment of Residential Care Homes on Dementia Suffers in Hong Kong: A Critical Incident Technique Approach," *Building and Environment* 73 (2014): 32–39.

72 John Zeisel, Nina M. Silverstein, Joan Hyde, S. Sue Levkoff, M. Powell Lawton, and William Holmes, "Environmental Correlates to Behavioral Health Outcomes in Alzheimer's Special Care Units," *The Gerontologist* 43, no. 5 (2003): 697–711.

73 T. Anne Cleary, Cheryll Clamon, Marjorie Price, and Gail Shullaw, "A Reduced Stimulation Unit: Effects on Patients With Alzheimer's Disease and Related Disorders," *The Gerontologist* 28, no. 4 (1988): 511–514.

74 Emily Roberts, "Six for Lunch: A Dining Option for Residents With Dementia in a Special Care Unit," *Journal of Housing For the Elderly* 25, no. 4 (2011): 352–379.

4

DESIGNING TO CONFRONT THE ADVERSE HEALTH IMPACTS OF WORKPLACE SITTING

Takemi Sugiyama, Neville Owen, and Lynne M. Dearborn

Introduction

Prolonged time spent sitting is a newly identified health risk. Given that much of adults' daily sitting time is accrued in office workplace contexts, there is a need to better understand the sitting-related attributes of these indoor environments in which working adults may spend a majority of their waking hours. We highlight new evidence from epidemiological and experimental research demonstrating that prolonged uninterrupted sitting, as distinct from doing too little exercise, can increase the risk of obesity, type 2 diabetes, cardiovascular disease, and some cancers. Reducing sedentary behaviors is now a preventive-health priority, for which a better understanding of the design factors that may influence sitting in these indoor environments is needed.

Thus, our agenda for this chapter is to introduce a perspective that we hope will help to identify new opportunities for research and practice in workplace design. To do so, we first introduce the "behavior settings" construct from ecological psychology, which emphasizes how the attributes of environments can mandate or promote certain behaviors and discourage others. In this context, we then suggest the utility of "routes" and "destinations" as behavior-setting attributes with potential influence on length of time spent in seated activities. We provide examples from recent research studies and consider how these may function at the micro-scale of indoor workplace environments.

In this context, we propose interdisciplinary research collaborations involving epidemiology, behavioral science, and architectural design[1] that can help to refine current thinking and provide new evidence with the potential to inform innovative approaches to workplace design.

Health Impacts of Prolonged Sitting

The importance of regularly engaging in combinations of moderate-intensity and vigorous-intensity physical activity and planned exercise to maintain good health and reduce risk of premature mortality from the major chronic diseases (i.e., type 2 diabetes, heart disease, several cancers) and a range of other health problems is now well understood. Exercising and physical activities that confer important health benefits include not only vigorous-intensity exercise such as jogging and swimming (greatly increasing heart rate) but also moderate-intensity activity such as brisk walking and cycling.[2]

However, people can be physically active in these ways, but can also spend prolonged periods of time sitting: especially at work, in automobiles, and at home. Prolonged periods of time spent in these sedentary behaviors—put simply, too much sitting as distinct from too little exercise—are now known to increase chronic disease risk and are newly-developing elements of national preventive-health agendas.[3]

Reducing overall workplace sitting time and promoting frequent, brief interruptions to sitting time has considerable potential to provide widespread health benefits.[4] In this context, reducing workers' exposures to environmental attributes that mandate or promote prolonged, unbroken periods of sitting time is a new public health imperative.[5] Environmental design has much to offer in these examinations of sitting time and in the explorations of how best to appropriately interrupt extensive periods of sitting in the workplace.

A Large Amount of Adults' Sitting Time Occurs in the Work Environment

Sitting occurs in different behavior settings: at home (domestic), at work, commuting between home and work, and in the community where one lives. In particular, office environments are generally associated with extensive sitting time for working adults. Studies find that office workers spend around two-thirds to three-quarters of their average work day in sitting and other sedentary behaviors.[6] Among desk-based workers, sitting at work constituted more than 50 percent of total daily sitting time.[7] Figure 4.1, based on findings from a British survey of working adults, illustrates the high proportion of daily sitting time that can be accumulated in the office workplace setting. Domestic and commuting settings (i.e., vehicles) also account for a significant amount of daily sitting time. The striped portions in the outer concentric ring in Figure 4.1 suggest the limited options for individual-level change. However, a comparison of the outer concentric ring's stripped portion to its solid portion, particularly that associated with the work setting, indicates the broad opportunity area where design initiatives could influence a reduction in sitting time and a change toward healthier patterns of sitting.[8]

Many studies of workplace behavior suggest that sitting at work, which adds substantially to overall sedentary time for adult office workers, is a very common behavior that merits attention. Since high levels of overall sitting time and unbroken periods of sitting are associated with an increased risk of developing cardiometabolic as well as musculoskeletal problems,[9] design initiatives that target the reduction of occupational sitting have considerable, and as yet unrealized, potential for enhancing workers' health.

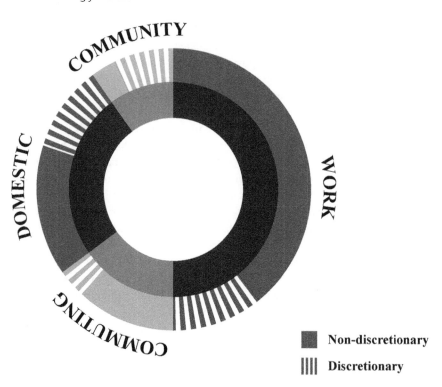

FIGURE 4.1   Primary Behavior Settings Where Sitting Time Accrues and Potential for Discretionary Reductions

Environmental Initiatives to Reduce Workplace Sitting

In light of a growing concern about workplace sitting, research has begun to examine various approaches to reduce sitting time. A recent review found that interventions to reduce workplace sitting focusing on educational or behavioral approaches (e.g., providing information about health impacts of prolonged sitting; goal setting; self-monitoring) often produce non-significant or small effects.[10] In contrast, the same review reported that environmental interventions yielded a significant and larger reduction in sitting time. The importance of settings where behaviors take place is consistent with an ecological model, in which multi-level (individual, environmental, and social) approaches are considered to be effective in facilitating behavior change.[11]

An ecological model of the workplace behavior setting, illustrated in Figure 4.2, examined with respect to sedentary behaviors, emphasizes the central role of those physical-environment and social/organizational attributes of the contexts in which people spend significant numbers of their waking hours. While acknowledging the relevance of individual-level attributes such as awareness of health risks and motivation to change, the primary emphasis of the ecological model is on how the attributes of the settings in which people spend their time can mandate or promote

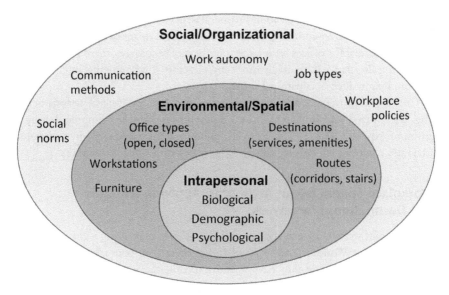

FIGURE 4.2 An Ecological Model of the Workplace Behavior Setting Identifying Factors Across Nested Scales that May Influence Sitting Activity Patterns

Source: This figure draws from Neville Owen, et al., "Adults' Sedentary Behavior," *American Journal of Preventive Medicine*, 41, no. 2. (August 2011): 191.

certain behaviors and discourage other behaviors. Applying the ecological model of sedentary behavior to occupational settings, in particular to office environments in which so many workers spend a high proportion of their working hours sitting, provides a compelling case in point for such environmental effects.

An ecological perspective on designing to confront the adverse health outcomes of workplace sitting (see Figure 4.2) acknowledges that components of both the physical-environmental and social-organizational contexts join with individual motivations and preferences to influence sitting patterns and overall time spent in such sedentary behaviors in the workplace. There is the need to focus on particular contexts within which particular behaviors take place in order to understand the most effective environmental-change initiatives to disperse and limit episodes of sedentary behavior.[12] Examining the nested scales identified in this model highlights the importance of specific physical-environment elements that can be modified through design to affect and reduce sedentary workplace behaviors, thus confronting adverse health outcomes of workplace sitting through environmental design. Likewise, it emphasizes that physical-environment modifications will likely be most effective in combination with social/organizational strategies that also acknowledge individual level worker attributes.

Office-environment factors and characteristics that promote sitting can be amenable to change. For example, environmental interventions to reduce occupational sitting currently focus on installation of equipment that enables standing or lower limb movement, particularly height-adjustable, stationary-cycle, and treadmill desks.

Such interventions have been found to be effective, but obviously work only for those who have the equipment. Given that they involve financial investment, which can be substantial for offices with larger numbers of employees, there is a scope for developing alternative (potentially more cost effective) environmental interventions that can help reduce occupational sitting.

Creating a "movement-friendly" workplace in which prolonged periods of sitting are reduced and broken up more frequently is indeed recommended by a group of experts.[13] However, it is as yet unknown what workplace environmental attributes can most effectively influence the sitting time of office workers.

Workplace Spatial-layout Attributes: Applying a Routes and Destinations Framework

An important setting characteristic within the office is that sitting is the normal or default behavior. Workers tend to sit whenever there is an opportunity, and sitting is interrupted only when they have to move to other areas within the workplace. Thus, sitting and movement within the workplace are likely to be determined to a significant extent by the spatial arrangement of locations in which various functions and tasks are to be performed. The study of workplace spatial factors that might facilitate more movement and less sitting can be informed by an established body of research on neighborhood environments and physical activity. Research on neighborhood environmental correlates of physical activity has progressed substantially over last two decades; it now produces specific evidence that informs urban planning policy.[14]

A conceptual framework of "destinations and routes," used to analyze neighborhood walking behavior,[15] has potential applicability for workplace environments as well. In the case of neighborhoods, destinations can refer to local shops, cafés, and transport stops, while routes are streets and paths to get to such destinations.

At the local-neighborhood scale, the attributes of destinations and routes are known to be associated with residents' physical activity. For instance, better access to and a greater mix of local destinations are associated with more frequent walking.[16] Route attributes such as street patterns and connectivity are also found to be related to walking.[17] Well-connected streets (often within grid-type street patterns) facilitate walking partly because they provide more direct access to destinations, compared to less connected streets (e.g., cul-de-sac), where travel distance can be longer due to street configuration.[18]

This conceptual model of routes and destinations can be applied at a smaller scale to identify relevant attributes of the workplace environment. These specific attributes can then be examined in multi-site observational studies and modified through design in follow-up experimental studies to test if they do in fact reduce and break up workers' sitting time. It may be hypothesized, for example, that workers who have more destinations within the workplace that are more easily accessed are more likely to be active and sit less. Destinations within the workplace might include service and amenity functions such as meeting places, printers/copiers, restrooms, kitchen/meal areas, and elevators, while routes include circulation space such as corridors and staircases.

Destinations within Office Environment that Can Reduce and Break Up Sitting

A recent study showed associations among the distance to services and amenities with walking step totals logged by office workers; participants who had shared functions (meeting room, copy area, kitchen, reception, and elevator) nearby walked more than those who had them farther from their workstation.[19] Since the study measured the number of steps walked, the findings suggest that those who had the service/amenity areas nearby would have spent more of their work time walking, through more frequent visits to these destinations.

This interpretation is supported by an innovative study using an indoor tracking system, which showed that workers' movement (the number of steps) while at the office was associated with the number of trips they made to destinations such as the kitchen and the desks of other people.[20] These findings suggest that offices may not have to be large to reduce sitting time and facilitate more movement. An office cluster with necessary functions that are shared by a relatively small number of workers may facilitate more movement within the workplace than can business environments with areas dedicated to larger clusters of offices. These findings also suggest that availability of such destinations in the workplace could break up prolonged sitting, which is known to be relevant to health, independent of overall sitting time.[21] Thus, research might investigate the size of an office cluster that can minimize workplace sitting.

However, interestingly, another workplace study did not find any association between proximity to functions and sedentary time.[22] Since this study used accelerometers to measure sedentary time, it may have counted time spent standing (e.g., at meeting room, copy area, kitchen) as sedentary, which may have contributed to non-significant associations. Using the indoor tracking system, Spinney and colleagues found that one trip to the kitchen on average involved eight minutes of standing per hour.[23] Further research on workplace destinations and sitting using more accurate measures (e.g., inclinometer attached to each participant's thigh) is warranted.

Routes within Office Environment that Can Reduce and Break Up Sitting

At the micro-scale of the workplace, routes may be well-defined in the case of enclosed offices (or those with high partitions), but may be less so in the case of open office (with low or no partitions). Regardless of such differences, how routes are configured within the workplace may influence workers' movement and sitting.

An Australian study, for example, examined associations of connectivity of routes (based on self-reported assessment of how routes intersect each other and availability of multiple routes to destinations) with the number of breaks in sitting. Having more connected routes was negatively associated with total sitting time and positively associated with the number of breaks. This study also found that those who reported clear visual access to a colleague's desk broke their sitting time more often than those who reported less clear visual access.[24]

It may be argued that visual access to various functions (or possibly other workers' activities) may be relevant. An experimental study observing the change of workers' behaviors before and after moving to a new office, which featured open meeting spaces and highly visible staircases as well as height-adjustable desks, found after the move a significant increase in standing time and a decrease in sitting time that approached statistical significance.[25] Research evidence on the relationship between route configuration and within-office movement requires greater clarity to provide useful design guidance. However, these initial findings seem to suggest that physical and visual access to various functions may play a role in workplace behavior.

Future Research Directions

Research on workplace environments and workers' sitting is in its early stages. Evidence from prior research on neighborhood environments and physical activity (along with early evidence on workplaces) appears to indicate the importance of spatial arrangement of office functions. However, further research is needed to advance our understanding of workplace attributes that can enhance workers' health. Additional focus in a number of possible future research areas, identified below, will yield important advances regarding the design of workplace environments and sedentary behaviors.

There is a need for research to examine specific attributes of destinations and routes. Hua and Yang explored the distance to destinations within the workplace.[26] It is plausible that other attributes of destinations, such as size, quality, and visual access, can influence the use of these spaces. Access to "external" destinations, such as outdoor spaces and shops, may also prove relevant to the pattern of workplace sitting. For routes, in addition to connectivity, attributes such as width, outside views, and presence of a space for "corridor-talk" may also be pertinent.

Future research focused on ways to reduce sedentary behavior in the office environment through design initiatives needs to develop new measurement techniques and to conduct controlled studies, especially so in the evaluation of "natural experiments" provided by innovative workplace design initiatives. Also, studies should include large sample sizes and different participant populations (for example, call-center workers or office-based professionals), and also develop new tools to assess and compare physical features of the environment.

Several "natural experiments" observing behaviors before and after moving to a new office have been reported. However, they are small in scale (less than 50 participants), and not able to quantify the differences between the old and new workplace environments.[27] To better understand what workplace attributes can contribute most strongly to sedentary behavior changes, it is particularly important to develop instruments that can assess physical and social office environmental factors in a quantitative manner.

To change the general mindset concerning office behavior settings, economic evaluations of workplace innovations are needed. To convince employers (and, particularly in the United States, developers of office space) to produce movement-friendly physical environments, research evaluating their economic benefits needs to be conducted. Workplace productivity is challenging to measure, but indicators such as sick leave may be used to assess cost savings due to movement-friendly design.

The ecological perspective on workplace sitting illustrated in Figure 4.2 highlights the additional importance of organizational factors in the workplace setting. Whatever environmental-design initiatives are introduced, behavior choices within the workplace will be supported or constrained by organizational factors, such as social norms and regulations within the workplace.[28] Thus, availability of destinations may not necessarily mean more movement and less sitting if the organizational milieu does not permit free movement. Researchers need to develop measures for such factors and to test interventions to alter them.

Conclusions

Workplace design has conventionally focused on maximizing work efficiency through minimizing disruption by non-work related activities.[29] However, recent research now strongly suggests that office environments where workers are simply encouraged to sit in their workstation for a prolonged period will have broad-reaching adverse health impacts. Workplace design that sets out to explicitly promote more movement and less sitting holds great promise to provide much-needed preventive health solutions. Furthermore, better health among workers enhances productivity by reducing sick leave and absenteeism. For United States-based employers who contribute to health insurance premiums, better physical and mental health among workers may translate into a reduction in premiums overall.

In addition, a workplace that facilitates workers' movement through well-connected routes can generate more face-to-face interactions, which could support collaboration, enhance the office social climate, and improve workers' mental health.[30] However, it is also important to be aware of potentially negative aspects of such workplace design; movement-friendly office environments may have unintended consequences that increase worker stress due to noise, perceived lack of privacy, and crowded conditions.

Further research examining specific workplace attributes that encourage more movement and less sitting is warranted to help architects and interior designers make informed design decisions. The ecological model presented in this chapter, as well as the numerous studies referenced, provide a robust starting point for researchers and designers to build collaborations that can lead to a new and substantial body of knowledge within which the health impacts of environmental design may be addressed. Findings from studies of health–workplace–design links might also spur thought and debate that is relevant to the design of other of environment types (e.g., school settings, residential environments, and entertainment venues).

University educational initiatives in health and design will be particularly important in this context. Those responsible for design and health teaching programs may find our framework, presented earlier, helpful in building more explicit and more comprehensive links between design, human behavior, and health. The ubiquitous nature of sitting at work and in many other environments—now that health risks are becoming increasingly clear—provides a compelling case in point with a plethora of opportunities for interdisciplinary teaching, design innovation, and associated collaborations in research. Public Health, Epidemiology, Physical Therapy, Psychology, Sociology, Architecture, Interior Design, and Occupational Health come to mind as some of the key partnerships for interdisciplinary design and health teaching and research.

We hope that we have illustrated in this chapter the potential value of an *ecological model* and a *routes and destinations* framework to help account for the determinants of sitting behavior in the workplace and possibly for other physical-environmental contexts where people spend many of their waking hours. There is considerable capacity for many new design initiatives that will help greatly to address *too much sitting* as a ubiquitous health risk

Notes

1 Weimo Zhu and Neville Owen, *Sedentary Behavior and Health: Concepts, Evidence, Assessment and Intervention* (Urbana-Champaign: Human Kinetics, 2016).
2 William L. Haskell et al., "Physical Activity and Public Health: Updated Recommendation for Adults From the American College of Sports Medicine and the American Heart Association," *Circulation* 116 (2007): 1081–1093.
3 I-Min Lee et al., "Effect of Physical Inactivity on Major Non-Communicable Diseases Worldwide: An Analysis of Burden of Disease and Life Expectancy," *The Lancet* 380, no. 9838 (2012): 219–229; Takemi Sugiyama et al., "Adverse Associations of Car Time with Markers of Cardio-Metabolic Risk," *Preventive Medicine* 83 (2016): 26–30.
4 Genevieve N. Healy et al., "Replacing Sitting Time With Standing or Stepping: Associations With Cardio-Metabolic Risk Biomarkers," *European Heart Journal* 36, no. 39 (October 2015): 2643–2649; Ulf Ekelund et al., "Does Physical Activity Attenuate the Detrimental Association of Sitting Time With Mortality?" *The Lancet* 388, no. 10051 (2016) : 1302–1310.
5 Neville Owen et al., "Adults' Sedentary Behavior Determinants and Interventions," *American Journal of Preventative Medicine* 41, no. 2 (2011): 189–196; Neville Owen et al., "Sedentary Behaviour and Health: Mapping Environmental and Social Context to Underpin Chronic Disease Prevention," *British Journal of Sports Medicine* 48, no. 3 (2014).
6 Gemma C. Ryde et al., "Desk-Based Occupational Sitting Patterns: Weight-Related Health Outcomes," *Journal of Preventive Medicine* 45, no. 4 (2013): 448–452; Alicia A. Thorp et al., "Prolonged Sedentary Time and Physical Activity in Workplace and Non-Work Contexts," *International Journal of Behavioral Nutrition and Physical Activity* 9 (2012): 1–9.
7 Jason A. Bennie et al., "Total and Domain-Specific Sitting Time Among Employees in Desk-Based Work Settings in Australia," *Australian and New Zealand Journal of Public Health* 39, no. 3 (2015): 237–242.
8 Ambreen Kazi et al., "A Survey of Sitting Time Among UK Employees," *Occupational Medicine* 64 (2014): 497–502.

9 John P. Buckley et al., "The Sedentary Office: An Expert Statement on the Growing Case for Change Towards Better Health and Productivity," *British Journal of Sports Medicine* 49, no. 21 (2015): 1357–1362.

10 Anne H. Chu, Sheryl H. X. Ng, Chuen Seng Tan, Wah Win, David Koh, and Falk Müller-Riemenschneider, "A Systematic Review and Meta-Analysis of Workplace Intervention Strategies to Reduce Sedentary Time in White-Collar Workers," *Obesity Reviews* 17, no. 5 (2016): 467–481.

11 Nyssa Hadgraft, David Dunstan, and Neville Owen, "Models for Understanding Sedentary Behavior," in *Sedentary Behavior Epidemiology*, eds. Michael Leitzmann, C. Carmen Jochem, and Daniela Schmid (Forthcoming); James F. Sallis and Neville Owen, "Ecological Models of Health Behavior," in *Health Behavior Theory, Research, and Practice*, eds. Karen Glanz, Barbara K. Rimer, and K.Viswanath (San Francisco, CA: Jossey-Bass, 2015): 43–64.

12 Owen, "Adults' Sedentary."

13 Buckley, "Sedentary Office."

14 Billie Giles-Corti et al., "Translating Active Living Research Into Policy and Practice," *Journal of Public Health Policy* 36, no. 2 (2015): 231–243.

15 Takemi Sugiyama et al., "Destination and Route Attributes Associated With Adults Walking," *Medicine and Science in Sports and Exercise* 44, no. 7 (2012): 1275–1286.

16 Tania L. King et al., "Does the Presence and Mix of Destinations Influence Walking and Physical Activity?" *International Journal of Behavioral Nutrition and Physical Activity* 12, no. 1 (2015): 1–12.

17 Wesley E. Marshall and Norman W. Garrick, "Effect of Street Network Design on Walking and Biking," *Transportation Research Record* 2198 (2010): 103–115.

18 David Berrigan, Linda W. Pickle, and Jennifer Dill, "Associations Between Street Connectivity and Active Transportation," *International Journal of Health Geographics* 9, no. 1 (2010): 1–20.

19 Ying Hua and Eunhwa Yang, "Building Spatial Layout That Supports Healthier Behavior of Office Workers," *Work* 49, no. 3 (2014): 373–380.

20 Richard Spinney et al., "Indoor Tracking to Understand Physical Activity and Sedentary Behaviour," *PLoS One* 10 (2015): 5.

21 Genevieve N. Healy et al., "Sedentary Time and Cardio-Metabolic Biomarkers in US Adults: NHANES 2003–06," *European Heart Journal* 32, no. 5 (2011): 590–597.

22 Hua, "Spatial Layout."

23 Spinney, "Indoor Tracking," 5.

24 Mitch J. Duncan et al., "Identifying Correlates of Breaks in Occupational Sitting," *Building Research & Information* 43, no. 5 (2015): 646–658.

25 Erin Gorman et al., "Does an 'Activity-Permissive' Workplace Change Office Workers Sitting and Activity Time?" *PLoS One* 8 (2013): 10.

26 Hua, "Spatial Layout."

27 Gorman, "Activity-Permissive," 2; Jonine Jancy et al., "Workplace Building Design and Office-Based Workers' Activity," *Australian and New Zealand Journal of Public Health* 40, no. 1 (2016): 78–82.

28 Genevieve N. Healy et al., "Reducing Sitting Time in Office Workers," *Preventive Medicine* 57, no. 1 (2013): 2643–2649.

29 Hua, "Spatial Layout."

30 Jean Wineman et al., "Spatial and Social Networks in Organizational Innovation,' *Environment and Behavior* 41, no. 3 (2009):) : 427–442.

5

COMMUNICABLE DISEASES AND OUR ENVIRONMENTS

Robin Toft Klar and Susan O'Hara

Introduction

The connection between communicable disease and the environment was understood by very observant clinicians well before germ theory was discovered and put into practice. Translating the sciences of microbiology and epidemiology into the design of environments has progressed as our understanding of these connections has evolved. Gone are the days of siloed knowledge development and practice. Health care providers (HCPs) are working together with architects, designers, engineers, and construction professionals to create effective and efficient residential and health care facilities that improve quality outcomes and safety for patients, clinicians, family members, and other visitors to wherever the patient is situated. This chapter will present descriptions of infectious diseases, their mode(s) of transmission, and how design can potentially interrupt the transmission of select communicable diseases. We will discuss the consequences of ignoring mode of disease transmission in design and techniques for considering infectious disease potential with each design idea and product. We will use the authors' developed framework of PROTECTED (Population, Resources, Observation/Surveillance, Transfer, Efficiency/Efficacy, Contagion, Transparency, Education, and Design) to present a means of gathering necessary information when considering communicable diseases, the environment, and its design's influence.

The Problem

Quality outcomes and the safety of patients and others have become the priority for the entire health care team. This is especially relevant when we are discussing communicable/infectious diseases. The burden of communicable diseases is felt in lives lost and disability as a consequence. Disability adjusted life years (DALY's) is a frequent measure of burden of disease. Approximately a quarter (23 percent) of global deaths are attributable to segments of the environment that are modifiable.[1] Those deaths resulting from communicable diseases include 57 million from diarrheal infections, 52 million from lower respiratory infections, and 23 million from malaria. The percentages of these deaths attributable to modifiable environments are 58 percent, 35 percent, and 42 percent, respectively. Modifications most frequently attributed to these deaths are water and sanitation, followed by housing improvements related to dense indoor settings.[2]

Actions required to decrease the spread of communicable diseases start with understanding the epidemiologic triangle which consists of agent, host, and environment. The agent refers to the organism responsible for the communicable disease. The host here is humans. The environment consists of natural and built environment factors that inhibit or permit the transmission of the agent to the host. All interventions, chemical (pharmaceuticals in the form of vaccines and antimicrobial medications and insecticides) or barrier (physical distance, personal protective equipment [PPE], and other barrier mechanisms), are attempts to break the chain of transmission. Understanding the mode or ways that the agent is transmitted to humans allows for design interventions to break the chain.

Infectious Diseases

The infectious diseases presented here are those that contribute the greatest burden of disease and/or have identified modifiable environmental design interventions. A theme will become apparent in this presentation of infectious diseases between the mode(s) of transmission and the design interventions to inhibit the transmission of bacteria, viruses, fungi, and protozoa.

Pneumonia

Pneumonia is a disease of the respiratory tract. The pneumococcal microbe (bacteria, virus, or fungus) is aerosolized by droplets originating from the nose or throat of one human and inhaled into the lungs of another human. Pneumonia can eventually move to other parts of the body and cause severe complications and/or death. Globally, pneumonia is the leading infectious disease responsible for the deaths of children 5 years and younger. In the U.S., pneumonia is more prevalent in the adult population, responsible for one million hospitalizations annually.[3] A recent retrospective cohort study identified a shift in the population and contagion of those occupying intensive care unit (ICU) beds in the U.S. Between 1996 and 2010 the age of elderly ICU patients increased and the primary diagnosis shifted from non-communicable disease, primarily coronary artery disease, to sepsis which accounted for 10.2 percent of admissions. Admission for respiratory diseases rose from 7.0 percent to 9.2 percent within this same time span.[4] No matter what may be influencing this shift in disease burden, intensive care units primarily designed for non-communicable diseases must rethink how functional the design of the units are with more infectious diseases being present. The design must consider the patients and the mode of transmission of the infectious disease and also protection of health care staff and visitors in these more often denser clinical spaces.

Influenza

Influenza is an upper respiratory illness caused by two types of influenza virus, Type A and Type B. It is found throughout the world and is highly contagious, spreading by droplet from as far away as 6 feet when people cough, sneeze, or talk. The virus may also spread by direct contact by touching a surface where the virus droplets have landed and then putting that hand to eyes, nose, or mouth. The influenza virus can be spread before the individual feels sick. The importance in preventing the spread of influenza is that influenza-related complications can lead to bacterial pneumonia which can have a very high mortality rate for vulnerable populations including children, elders, and those whose immune systems are compromised due to chronic diseases.

Preparation for the 2009 H1N1 Seasonal Influenza Pandemic brought emergency preparedness and design elements together in an effort to keep the transmission and morbidity of influenza lower than anticipated. Use of barrier methods such as screens and curtains in health care facilities and installation of hand sanitizing dispensers in public buildings contributed to lower morbidity from H1N1 influenza.[5]

Tuberculosis (TB)

Tuberculosis (TB) is an infectious disease caused by *Mycobacterium tuberculosis* and is spread by air through coughing, sneezing, or talking. TB can be present in other body organs; however, it is only infectious if it is in the lungs. The mycobacterium may remain latent for a short period of time or years. Once the body's immune system is compromised, due to an acute or chronic condition, the bacteria may become active and cause symptoms. It is this symptom-free latency period that has increased the incidence of TB in the U.S. Approximately two-thirds of TB cases in the U.S. are in foreign-born residents. The most effective way to decrease the incidence of TB in the U.S. is to increase surveillance and prevention in those countries from which the highest percentage of U.S. foreign-born residents originate.[6] Surveillance involves screening those who work in high risk areas such as health care providers and also those who have been in close contact with a patient with active TB. Prevention strategies include controlling the flow of air.

Escherichia coli (E. coli)

Escherichia coli (E. coli) is an infectious disease caused by strains in this large category of *Escherichia coli*. There are healthy strains of these bacteria in the lower intestinal tract; however, some forms of E. coli can cause disease. The most frequent strain of

E. coli is Shiga toxin-producing *E. coli* often referred to as *E. coli1057*. The mode of transmission for *E. coli1057* is by direct contact with animal or human feces. This usually occurs when the source of feces comes into contact with the mouth and is swallowed. Culprits include unpasteurized dairy products, fruits and vegetables that have not been properly cleaned with potable water, and consumption of foods prepared by someone who has not properly washed their hands after toileting. Symptoms include diarrhea and vomiting so further transmission is highly likely if proper hygiene does not occur between the ill person and others that they may come into contact with around food preparation or animal management. Prevention starts with proper hand washing and not ingesting unpasteurized products. Access to safe, potable water for proper hand washing is the most important environmental design intervention to target *E. coli1057*.[7]

Methicillin-Resistant Staphylococcus Aureus (MRSA)

Methicillin-resistant *Staphylococcus aureus* (MRSA) is a *Staphylococcus aureus* (staph) bacteria that cannot be treated with traditional antibiotics. MRSA is found both in health care settings and the community. Both are transmitted the same way via direct contact with the debris from a wound infected with staph. It is more insidious in the community because the general public is not as tuned in to the transfer of staph from contact via sharing personal items, human contact with someone who has a wound, or contact with someone who has recently been in a health care facility (employee, patient, or visitor).[8]

Ebola Virus Disease (EVD)

Ebola Virus Disease (EVD) is a virus of the Filoviridae family, genus *Ebolavirus*. This rare communicable disease has become widely known due to the recent EVD epidemic in West Africa. The virus is transmitted, initially, from an animal host, primarily fruit bats or primates, to humans. Once the virus is within the human host, it is transmitted by direct contact with bodily fluids or objects that have been in contact with EVD body fluids, such as needles, syringes, bandages, clothing, and condoms, to name a few. Prevention of EVD from animal hosts involves avoidance of contact with bats and not eating bush meat due to the high likelihood of it being infected with EVD. Prevention of human-to-human transmission involves strict adherence to using barrier methods to avoid contact with suspicious or actual EVD infected bodily secretions which include blood, urine, saliva, sweat, feces, vomit, breast milk, and semen.[9]

HIV/AIDS

HIV/AIDS is a one-two punch communicable disease that begins with the transmission of the human immunodeficiency virus (HIV) from human to human via direct contact with blood and body fluids containing HIV. Unlike most other viruses that enter the human body, HIV cannot be eliminated from the body after the virus runs its course. There is no vaccine currently available to prevent HIV; however, there are antiretroviral medications that can be taken as antiretroviral therapy (ART) to keep the virus in check and allow the patient to live a nearly normal life with this chronic disease. With the advancement of ART fewer patients with HIV convert to acquired immunodeficiency syndrome (AIDS) which presents with opportunistic infections, those that occur due to a compromised immune system, and cancers and is the late stage of HIV.[10] The fundamental prevention measure to avoid transmission of HIV is to not come into direct contact with blood and body fluids. Using barrier methods is the only way for sexual partners and health care workers to decrease the risk of transmission. For sexual partners the barrier method is correct use of condoms. Health care providers use gloves, masks, eye protection, and gowns to avoid any splash that might occur. This equipment is known as personal protective equipment (PPE) and not only must PPE be applied (donned) in the proper order it must be removed (doffed) in the proper order to avoid transmission with splashed fluids on the PPE.

Vaccine Preventable Infectious Diseases

Vaccine preventable infectious diseases are a category of communicable disease where the transmission of disease can be stopped with the administration of vaccines. There are currently 26 identified communicable diseases that can be prevented by vaccines. Immunizing the general public against these 26 communicable diseases creates a herd immunity for the whole population. Herd immunity provides protection to those who for various reasons do not receive immunizations. Depending on the vaccine there may be multiple doses, spaced at varying intervals to provide immunity. There are some vaccines that must be administered annually because the virus strains present in the general community change from year to year. The seasonal influenza vaccine is one such vaccine. Measles is an example of a communicable disease with a stable vaccine, combined with mumps and rubella (MMR), that has received attention recently due to a trend to not vaccinate children. This is a highly contagious disease that is spread by being in the same room with someone who has measles who breathes, coughs, or sneezes. The virus can remain virulent, able to transmit disease, for two hours after the infected person leaves the room.[11]

Malaria

Malaria is a serious, sometimes fatal, communicable disease transmitted by mosquitoes. Malaria is mostly found in tropical regions of the globe, sub-Saharan Africa, Latin America, and Asia. Malaria was responsible for 627,000 deaths globally in 2012, primarily young children.[12] If mosquitoes bite humans infected with malaria the parasites from humans can be transmitted to the mosquito continuing the agent/host cycle of the epidemiologic triangle. With the rapid speed of airline transportation infected mosquitoes can be trapped on airplanes and infect passengers who have not traveled to malaria endemic geographic areas of the globe that always have a certain level of disease. Malaria is an exemplar case of communicable diseases transmitted by mosquito.

Mosquito Transmitted Diseases

Mosquito transmitted diseases, the largest vector of vector-borne transmitted diseases, are responsible for one million deaths annually around the globe. More familiar mosquito transmitted diseases, in addition to malaria, include Chikungunya, Dengue, Yellow Fever, Eastern Equine Encephalitis, Western Equine Encephalitis, West Nile Virus, and Zika virus.[13] There is an effective vaccine for Yellow Fever and countries where Yellow Fever is endemic will not allow visitors entrance unless they show documentation of Yellow Fever vaccination.

Antibiotic Resistance

Antibiotic resistance is a public health issue around the globe. Staph, malaria, and TB are just a few of the communicable diseases that are resurging as a result of inappropriate use of antibiotics or not completing the full course of antibiotic treatment. The fundamental means to decrease antibiotic resistant diseases is to prevent the transmission of these diseases. There are two primary strategies that prevent the transmission of communicable disease: barriers and improved air quality. Physical barriers include gloves, gowns, facemasks, eye protection, occlusive dressings, condoms, lids on barrels of water, safety syringes, and used needle boxes. Chemical barriers include mosquito/vector repellant, vaccines, and antiretroviral therapy (ART). Improved air quality includes various filters, respirators, and expanding space to decrease density.

Implications for Design

Communicable diseases are found in populations (a group of people) who reside in communities with specific geographic boundaries. Some communities have invisible physical boundaries such as continents, countries, states, cities, or towns, while other communities have a more visible boundary such as residential, commercial, academic, or health care settings.

For the purposes of this chapter we will be discussing communicable diseases and design implications within congregate and health care settings. Congregate or shared housing settings include residences that are based on life choices such as military barracks or hardships such as correctional facilities, homeless shelters, and refugee camps. Others are based on health conditions such as nursing homes or rehabilitation centers (whether short-term or disease-specific). Some congregate housing is for special or seasonal events such as the Olympic village, or day and overnight camps. Design regulations are based on regulations of congregate housing and health care facilities. This definition of congregate housing is determined by the WHO,[14] while the Housing and Urban Development (HUD) authority definition includes low-income housing and campuses where residents congregate to have meals.[15]

Design and health care professionals work together to bring regulations, standards, and guidelines into the design and building of all settings to prevent disease from transferring and to protect the members of that community. These professionals include architects, planners, and engineers using the national guidelines such the Facility Guidelines Institute,[16] American Society of Heating, Refrigeration, and Air Conditioning Engineers (ASHRAE),[17] and Occupational Safety and Health Administration (OSHA).[18] Some of these guidelines and standards are state specific such as in California. In this state the Office of Statewide Health Planning and Development (OSHPD) focuses on building health care institutions and provides data and construction guidelines.[19] Each state also has a department of public health, which provides standards for building health care institutions. These standards bridge the design and construction industry with the health care industry.

In the health care industry there are global, national, and public regulatory and educational resources put forward to offer prevention and management of disease. Internationally, the World Health Organization (WHO) is charged with this work.[20] In the U.S., the Centers for Disease Control and Prevention (CDC) is a federal agency that provides data and guidelines on all disease conditions,[21] while the American Public Health Association advocates prevention and promotion of health for the community.[22]

This section will draw from these agencies for overall information and move to disease-specific standards. In the residence and congregate home setting handwashing and use of personal protection equipment (PPE) have been found to be beneficial. In health care facilities, design of private rooms, improved ventilation, and finishes and surfaces have helped to decrease the spread of disease.

Disease-Specific Design Implications

In this section we will organize design implications by methods of transmission. Airborne transmission of tuberculosis (TB) and droplet transmission of pneumonia and influenza will be discussed. Design implications for direct contact transmitted diseases including influenza, *Escherichia coli* (*E. coli*), methicillin-resistant *Staphylococcus aureus* (MRSA), Ebola, and human immunodeficiency virus/and human immunodeficiency virus infection and acquired immune deficiency syndrome (HIV/AIDs) are discussed. Mosquito borne illnesses such as malaria and Zika will also be discussed. Finally, another perspective called infection bundles completes this section.

Airborne Transmission

Airborne transmission of TB can be reduced by improving the quantity and quality of ventilation. TB and other organisms can be transmitted when the microorganisms causing these diseases pass through systems such as air-conditioning units, especially if the maintenance has been insufficient. If these air conditioning systems are in places where other persons have illnesses and have a weakened immune system, the airborne disease can spread to those persons. Measures to protect people from airborne organisms are similar to all communicable disease prevention: administrative, environmental, and PPE. We will focus on the environmental measures.

There are two kinds of ventilation: natural and artificial.[23] Natural ventilation can be achieved in residential settings letting in fresh air by opening doors, skylights, and windows. Design of larger windows and adding fans can improve the exchange of indoor and outdoor air. Being outdoors is also an advantage for the TB patient and the members of the household and allows for directional airflow allowing the infected person to be located near exhaust and non-infected persons near air.[24,25] In areas where mosquitoes can also cause harm, screens should be applied to these openings.

In most hospital settings it is not possible to open windows so artificial filtration and ventilation are important key aspects of environmental control. The CDC suggests primary and secondary controls: ventilation, dilution, and controlling airflow near the source and cleaning the air.[26] Filtration is accomplished by improving indoor air quality through the removal of particulates in two ways—using High Efficiency Particulate Air (HEPA) filters and ultraviolet germicidal irradiation (UVGI). A high efficiency (99.97 percent minimum) particulate air (HEPA) filter is used to improve air quality by filtering out aerosolized particles of 0.3 micrometers in diameter. Ultraviolet germicidal irradiation uses light waves to decrease communicable disease droplet transmission when located in either the upper room or in the HVAC system ducts.[27,28]

There is some controversy about the optimal ventilation system in the hospital setting.[29,30] What is known is that UVGI can augment the use of HEPA filters. A 90 percent efficient filter is adequate for most hospital settings and increasing to 99.97 percent HEPA filtrations can remove particles of 0.3 μm.[31] The CDC has published guidelines for use of UVGI in the TB environment.[32]

Specialized airborne infection control isolation rooms (AIIRS) require design implementations including ante-rooms, airflow pressure differences between the room, ante-room, and main unit or corridor, and additional exhaust mechanisms.[33,34] It is important to refer to CDC, ASHRAE, and FGI for details about these design regulations. Originally, guidelines for airborne infections focused on air changes per hour. However, current research is focused on directional airflow and ventilation between the source of disease (person) and the exhaust.[35,36] Separate spaces between persons who are both ill and not infected by making the transmission distances greater than 3 feet will decrease risk factors.[37]

Droplet Transmission

Design implications for pneumonia and influenza, transmitted by aerosolized droplets, is similar to airborne transmission design. In the case of pneumonia these droplets come from the nose or throat of the person with the disease and are inhaled into the lungs of the healthy person. In influenza this transmission occurs during talking, sneezing, and coughing. Other methods for transmitting organisms include feces atomized during flushing, or particles aerosolized during suctioning, intubation, and other procedures. Vomiting may also be a source of transmission.[38] Prevention using the infection control bundle approach makes sense in droplet transmission.

Design can be planned according to the size of the particle and the range of transmission, either short range or long range, and the path between the source and the exhaust.[39] Again, in using the prevention by infection control bundle we approach both the ventilation system and also the surfaces that these droplet nuclei have landed on.

Direct Contact Transmission

Influenza (surface to mouth and nose), *E. coli* (contact with human or animal feces), and MRSA (contact with personal items and wound infected with organism) are all preventable. The way to differentiate between contact transmission sources is to categorize by frequent and minimal hand contact. In frequent hand contact high touch surfaces such as doorknobs, medical equipment, light switches, bedrails, and more can be the source of transmission. In the hospital setting this can also include toilet and privacy curtain areas. Floors and ceilings are more often associated with minimal contact areas and this is found in products that promote fungi and bacterial growth and airborne transmission of these pathogens.

The most important design implication for direct contact transmission is increasing quantity and access to handwashing sinks. In the hospital setting, single-bed rooms with handwashing sinks and soap dispensers have decreased transmission of diseases.[40]

Design implications and implementation can be related to interior design features although some of these recent trends, such as the use of specially treated paints and carpets, have been refuted.[41]

The general approach besides handwashing sinks is to use vinyl surfaces instead of carpet and mechanical 'push plates'. Mesh material on chairs is more difficult to clean and should be reevaluated because organisms can survive on surfaces for many months.

Contact via phones and handheld devices are the latest problems in surface contact contamination based on the trend of electronic records and communication.[42]

In 2007 the CDC along with NIOSH (National Institute for Occupational Safety and Health) published guidelines to guide the overall core practices for prevention of transmission of infectious agents.[43] Use of PPE and handwashing as well as design features for sharps containers and other infectious waste (dressings, tissues, linen, etc.) should be readily accessible, visible, and adjacent to all areas the infected person occupies. Sinks and receptacles with no touch mechanisms should be designed, built, and implemented. In the health care setting or congregate housing, these precautions are to protect the patient, the HCPs and workers, the family and visitors, other residents, and ultimately the community.[44]

Mosquito Borne Diseases Transmission

This transmission can be averted through design and improved ventilation. In the residential setting, design is related to the stages of the mosquito life span. Begin with evaluation of the existing conditions of the home. Design to halt mosquito borne disease transmission is dependent on the life cycle of the mosquito. In the larvae stage there is a need for water to mature to adult mosquito. It is important to avoid water features and flat roofs and improve drainage of plant saucers, drain spouts, and gutters. In short no standing water should occur. If standing water cannot be eliminated, then design to cover the standing water and removal and replacement of that cover with easy motion is important. Once the mosquito is an adult, design features should focus on keeping the mosquitoes away from humans. These features include installing screens and adding fans to move mosquitoes through the air.

A variety of materials have been used to form a barrier to the mosquito that transmits malaria. The most frequent barrier system, especially in low and middle income countries, is insecticide treated synthetic netting. When possible, closing the eaves is effective for the entire building and not just the immediate space covered by a net.[45]

It is also important to note that mosquitoes fly close to the ground seeking heat and blood. By raising homes above the ground, disease transmitted by mosquitoes can be reduced.[46]

Infection Control Bundles

The concept of infection control bundles, offers a multi-interventional and inter-professional approach to treating and preventing communicable diseases. These improvements can occur between facilities and the community and within residential, academic, and health care settings. Several authors have identified infection control bundles for A/H1NI influenza and TB,[47] seasonal influenza,[48] *Clostridium difficile*,[49] influenza-like illnesses,[50] and MRSA;[51] several integrative reviews examine multiple studies and organisms.[52]

This approach takes into account co-morbidity and health care. For example, people may be bed-ridden, immuno-suppressed or compromised, on different medications, or have invasive equipment such as naso-gastric tubes, urinary or intravenous catheters in place. Thus, using infection control bundles offers a more comprehensive approach.

Common to these infection control bundles are administration, education, surveillance, prevention measures, and pharmacological interventions and audits. Environmental prevention and treatment can be sorted by processes, products and equipment, and design features.

- Processes: handwashing, wearing PPE, cleaning of all high and low contact surfaces, and terminal room cleaning.
- Products: PPE, soap and water, bleach solutions, respirators, HEPA filters, and UVGI units

- Design features: Single-bedded rooms, elevated buildings, screening, interior features such as vinyl instead of carpet.

It is important to think about the social isolation and stigma that comes with infection control procedures such as single bedrooms and quarantine (depending on the residential or health care setting). Quarantine is an isolation method keeping all exposed and those where exposure is in question physically separated from the general population. In the U.S., the Department of Health and Human Services has statutory authority to implement quarantine. As far back as the plague to current treatment of persons infected with, and exposed to Ebola, residents have had psychological and sociological problems with infection control measures even if they are based on sound scientific evidence. Careful consideration should be made to support persons isolated due to infection, especially in congregate settings. It is also important to separate items within a space, such as in a hospital room or family kitchen by the purpose or use of that space.[53] In other words, the questions should be asked: is the kitchen table used for dressing changes and meals; should the bathroom have clean supplies; where is the disposals/sharps container? Terminal disposal questions must also be considered—what to do with needles in a public restroom, or large waste in a landfill? However, these issues are outside the scope of this chapter.

"PROTECTED"

There are many factors to consider when designing residential and health care facilities with a focus on stopping or decreasing the transmission of infectious diseases. To remember the important features of infection control and design implications, we suggest using the mnemonic "PROTECTED", as seen in Table 5.1.

TABLE 5.1 PROTECTED Model Using TB Case for Design

	TUBERCULOSIS	*PROCESS*	*EQUIPMENT*	*ENVIRONMENT*
P	POPULATION	Identify at risk groups such as recent travelers from TB endemic regions of the globe and those living in congregate housing		Densely populated areas
R	RESOURCES	Health care providers (HCPs)	• Access to diagnostic procedures • PPE for HCPs	Health care facilities

	TUBERCULOSIS	PROCESS	EQUIPMENT	ENVIRONMENT
O	OBSERVATION/ SURVEILLANCE	• Direct Observation Therapy (DOT) • Surveillance	• Prescribed medication administration • PPE for HCP • National and regional data repositories	• Community or health care facility • Rapid communication between HCP and Public Health Departments
T	TRANSFER	Airborne, aerosolized	PPEs	Living in communities with high percentage of foreign-born residents or congregate housing
E	EFFICIENCY/ EFFICACY	Timely screening, diagnostic testing, and treatment	HCPs Skin, blood, and sputum testing, X-rays Prescribed medication	Use of lay and professional HCPs to go where client lives
C	CONTAGION	*Mycobacterium tuberculosis* aerosolized		Densely populated areas with high percentage of at-risk populations
T	TRANSPARENCY	• Notifying public about signs and symptoms • Easy communication of cases	Public service announcements (PSA) • Computers, smart phone apps • Predictive epidemiological and Geographic Information System analysis software	• Increased frequency and dissemination variety of PSAs in at-risk environments • Busy diagnostic and HCP settings
E	EDUCATION	Respiratory hygiene practices	Policy and procedures manuals	Disease-specific setting
D	DESIGN	• Interprofessional design team meetings • Environmental assessment	• Evidence-based guidelines	• Appropriate all equipment storage • Ventilation and filtration • Or = to 3 feet between infected non-infected • Negative pressure room as needed

Conclusion

In conclusion, as the completed PROTECTED table demonstrates, knowledge of the infective agent and mode of transmission of an infectious disease provides the designer with the ability to design specific barriers and air circulation products. There will continue to be new infectious diseases discovered or resurgences of neglected tropical and other lesser known diseases. However, as long as the inter-professional clinical and design teams of residential and health care clinical spaces remembers the epidemiologic triangle and why each component is important, transmission should be slowed or halted.

Notes

1 Annette Prüss-Üstün and Carlos Corvalán, *Preventing Disease Through Healthy Environments: Towards an Estimate of the Environmental Burden of Disease* (Geneva: World Health Organization, 2006).
2 Ibid.
3 Center for Disease Control and Prevention, "Pneumonia Can Be Prevented—Vaccines Can Help," www.cdc.gov/Features/Pneumonia/.
4 Michael W. Sjoding, Hallie C. Prescott, Hannah Wunsch, Theodore J. Iwashyna, and Colin R. Cooke, "Longitudinal Changes in ICU Admissions Among Elderly Patients in the United States," *Critical Care Medicine* 44, no. 7 (2016): 1353–1360.
5 Centers for Disease Control and Prevention, "Prevention Strategies for Seasonal Influenza in Healthcare Settings," www.cdc.gov/flu/professionals/infectioncontrol/healthcare settings.html.
6 Jorge L. Salinas, "Leveling of Tuberculosis Incidence—United States, 2013–2015," *MMWR: Morbidity and Mortality Weekly Report* 65 (2016): 273–278.
7 Centers for Disease Control and Prevention, "*E. coli* (*Escherichia coli*): General Information," www.cdc.gov/ecoli/general/index.html.
8 Centers for Disease Control and Prevention, "Methicillin-Resistant *Staphylococcous aureus*," www.cdc.gov/mrsa/index.html.
9 Centers for Disease Control and Prevention, "Ebola (Ebola Virus Disease)," www.cdc.gov/vhf/ebola/about.html.
10 Centers for Disease Control and Prevention, "HIV/AIDS," www.cdc.gov/hiv/basics/whatishiv.html.
11 Centers for Disease Control and Prevention, "Vaccines and Immunizations," www.cdc.gov/vaccines/vac-gen/why.html.
12 Centers for Disease Control and Prevention, "Malaria Worldwide," www.cdc.gov/malaria/malaria_worldwide/index.html.
13 American Mosquito Control Association, "Mosquito-Borne Diseases," www.mosquito.org/mosquito-borne-diseases#LAC.
14 World Health Organization, *WHO Policy on TB Infection Control in Health-Care Facilities, Congregate Settings and Households* (Geneva: World Health Organization, 2009).
15 Congregate Housing Services U.S. Codes § 8002 Title 42, The Public Health and Welfare, Chapter 89, http://energy.gov/sites/prod/files/2013/06/f1/doe-std-3020-2005.pdf.
16 Douglas S. Erickson, *Healthcare 101—FGI Primer*, in *Emerging Professionals Education Series—HC 101* (American Institute of Architects, 2015), http://network.aia.org/HigherLogic/System/DownloadDocumentFile.ashx?DocumentFileKey=6cba7c0e-caa0-4082-9093-76e2d61adfdc.
17 Lawrence J. Schoen, Michael J. Hodgson, William F. McCoy, Shelly L. Miller, Yuguo Li, and Russel N. Olmsted, "ASHRAE Position Document on Airborne Infectious Diseases," 2014, www.ashrae.org/standards-research—technology/standards—guidelines.

18 Occupational Health and Safety Administration, "Occupational Health and Safety Administration," www.osha.gov/.

19 State of California, "Office of Statewide Health and Planning Development," www.oshpd.ca.gov/.

20 World Health Organization, "About WHO," www.who.int/about/en/.

21 Centers for Disease Control and Prevention, "Centers for Disease Control and Prevention," www.cdc.gov/.

22 American Public Health Association, "American Public Health Association. For Science. For Action. For Health," www.apha.org/.

23 World Health Organization, "Health and Sustainable Development," www.who.int/sustainable-development/health-sector/health-risks/airborne-diseases/en/.

24 World Health Organization, "Policy on TB Infection," www.who.int/tb/publications/tb-facilities-policy/en/.

25 Francis J. Curry National Tuberculosis Center, *Tuberculosis Infection Control: A Practical Manual for Preventing TB* (San Francisco, CA: Curry National Tuberculosis Center, 2007).

26 Paul A. Jensen, Lauren A. Lambert, Michael F. Iademarco, Renee Ridzon, and Centers for Disease Control and Prevention, *Guidelines for Preventing the Transmission of Mycobacterium Tuberculosis in Health-Care Settings, 2005* (Hyattsville, M.D.: US Department of Health and Human Services, Public Health Service, Centers for Disease Control and Prevention, 2005).

27 James Atkinson, Yves Chartier, Carmen Lucia Pessoa Silvia, Paul Jensen, Yuguo Li, and Wing Hong Seto, eds. *Natural Ventilation for Infection Control in Health-Care Settings* (Geneva: World Health Organization, 2009).

28 U.S. Department of Energy, "Specification for HEPA Filters Used by DOE Contractors," DOE-STD-3020-97, 1997, http://energy.gov/sites/prod/files/2013/06/f1/doe-std-3020-2005.pdf.

29 Lynne Sehulster, Raymond Y.W. Chinn, Matthew J. Arduino, Joe Carpenter, Rodney Donlan, David Ashford, Richard Besser, et al., "Guidelines for Environmental Infection Control in Health-Care Facilities," *Morbidity and Mortality Weekly Report Recommendations and Reports RR* 52, no. 10 (2003): 1–48.

30 Craig Zimring, Anjali Joseph, and Ruchi Choudhary, *The Role of the Physical Environment in the Hospital of the 21st Century: A Once-in-a-Lifetime Opportunity* (Concord, CA: The Center for Health Design, 2004).

31 Sehulster, "Infection Control."

32 Centers for Disease Control and Prevention, "Environmental Control for Tuberculosis: Basic Upper-Room Ultraviolet Germicidal Irradiation Guidelines for Healthcare Settings," *Report No. DHHS (NIOSH) Publication* 2009-105 (2009).

33 Erickson, *FGI Primer*.

34 Schoen, "ASHRAE Position."

35 Ehsan S. Mousavi and Kevin R. Grosskopf, "Ventilation Rates and Airflow Pathways in Patient Rooms: A Case Study of Bioaerosol Containment and Removal," *Annals of Occupational Hygiene* 59, no.9 (2015): mev048.

36 Ehsan S. Mousavi and Kevin R. Grosskopf, "Directional Airflow and Ventilation in Hospitals: A Case Study of Secondary Airborne Infection," *Energy Procedia* 78 (2015): 1201–1206.

37 Peter Mendel, Sari Siegel, Kristin J. Leuschner, Elizabeth M. Gall, Daniel A. Weinberg, and Katherine L. Kahn, "The National Response for Preventing Healthcare—Associated Infections: Infrastructure Development," *Medical Care* 52 (2014): S17–S24.

38 Nicholas S. Holmes and Lidia Morawska, "A Review of Dispersion Modelling and Its Application to the Dispersion of Particles: An Overview of Different Dispersion Models Available," *Atmospheric Environment* 40, no. 30 (2006): 5902–5928.

39 Mousavi, "Ventilation Rates."

40 Anjali Joseph, *The Impact of the Environment on Infections in Healthcare Facilities* (Concord, CA: Center for Health Design, 2006).

41 Kaiser Permanente, "Kaiser Permanente Rejects Antimicrobials for Infection Control," https://share.kaiserpermanente.org/article/kaiser-permanente-rejects-antimicrobials-for-infection-control/.

42 Jaynelle F. Stichler, "Facility Design and Healthcare-Acquired Infections: State of the Science," *Journal of Nursing Administration* 44, no. 3 (2014): 129–132.

43 Jane D. Siegel, Emily Rhinehart, Marguerite Jackson, and Linda Chiarello, "2007 Guideline for Isolation Precautions: Preventing Transmission of Infectious Agents in Health Care Settings," *American Journal of Infection Control* 35, no. 10 (2007): S65–S164.

44 Emily S. Patterson, Jenna Murray, Sanghyun Park, Elizabeth B-N. Sanders, Jing Li, Radin Umar, Carolyn M. Sommerich, Kevin D. Evans, and Steven A. Lavender, "Barriers to Infection Control Due to Hospital Patient Room Factors: A Secondary Analysis of Focus Group and Interview Transcripts," in *Proceedings of the Human Factors and Ergonomics Society Annual Meeting* 58, no. 1 (Thousand Oaks, CA: Sage Publications, 2014): 1266–1270.

45 Steven W. Lindsay, Musa Jawara, K. Paine, Margaret Pinder, G. E. L. Walraven, and Paul M. Emerson, "Changes in House Design Reduce Exposure to Malaria Mosquitoes," *Tropical Medicine & International Health* 8, no. 6 (2003): 512–517.

46 Steve W. Lindsay, Paul M. Emerson, and J. Derek Charlwood, "Reducing Malaria By Mosquito-Proofing Houses," *Trends in Parasitology* 18, no. 11 (2002): 510–514.

47 Vincent C. C. Cheng, Joshua W. M. Tai, L. M. W. Wong, Jasper F. W. Chan, Iris W. S. Li, K. K. W. To, Ivan F. N. Hung, Koon Ho H. Chan, P. L. Ho, and Ky Yuen, "Prevention of Nosocomial Transmission of Swine-Origin Pandemic Influenza Virus A/H1N1 By Infection Control Bundle," *Journal of Hospital Infection* 74, no. 3 (2010): 271–277.

48 Pamela Hirsch, Michael Hodgson, and Victoria Davey, "Seasonal Influenza Vaccination of Healthcare Employees: Results of a 4-Year Campaign," *Infection Control & Hospital Epidemiology* 32, no. 5 (2011): 444–448.

49 Carlene A. Muto, Mary Kathleen Blank, Jane W. Marsh, Emanuel N. Vergis, Mary M. O'Leary, Kathleen A. Shutt, Anthony W. Pasculle, Marian Pokrywka, Juliet Garcia, Kathy Posey, Terri Roberts, Brian Potoski, Gary Blank, Richard Simmons, Peter Veldkamp, Lee Harrison, and David Patterson, "Control of an Outbreak of Infection With the Hyper-virulent Clostridium Difficile BI Strain in a University Hospital Using a Comprehensive 'Bundle' Approach," *Clinical Infectious Diseases* 45, no. 10 (2007): 1266–1273.

50 Anucha Apisarnthanarak, Piyaporn Apisarnthanarak, Boonsri Cheevakumjorn, and Linda M. Mundy, "Intervention With an Infection Control Bundle to Reduce Transmission of Influenza-Like Illnesses in a Thai Preschool," *Infection Control & Hospital Epidemiology* 30, no. 9 (2009): 817–822.

51 Gerd Fätkenheuer, Bernard Hirschel, and Stephan Harbarth, "Screening and Isolation to Control Meticillin-Resistant *Staphylococcus aureus*: Sense, Nonsense, and Evidence," *The Lancet* 385, no. 9973 (2015): 1146–1149.

52 Chantal Backman, Geoffrey Taylor, Anne Sales, and Patricia Beryl Marck, "An Integrative Review of Infection Prevention and Control Programs for Multidrug-Resistant Organisms in Acute Care Hospitals: A Socio-Ecological Perspective," *American Journal of Infection Control* 39, no. 5 (2011): 368–378.

53 Patterson, "Barriers to Infection Control."

6

ENVIRONMENTAL CONTAMINANTS

Amanda Hatherly

Introduction

Think of a home or building built 200 years ago. It was made of natural materials, (stone, adobe, wood, straw, etc.) and the people living in those buildings used natural materials for their clothing and cleaning. Doesn't it sound idyllic compared to the myriad of materials and chemicals we are exposed to today? Hold on! There were also fireplaces and stoves that exhausted combustion contaminants into the house and some of those building materials, such as asbestos and lead, were not as benign as that idyllic picture paints. In this chapter we are going to look at the reality of the indoor environment in buildings today, discuss the health impacts of those environments and look at how thoughtful design can make our homes and buildings healthier for us to inhabit. More and more evidence shows that our indoor environments impact our health, and careful design consideration can have a significant impact.

Common Interior Contaminants

Lead Paint

Lead is a highly toxic metal that, when absorbed into the bloodstream, causes damage to the brain, kidney, nerves and other vital organs. Lead may also cause learning disabilities and behavioral problems. In the past many buildings were painted with lead-based paint (which was banned in the U.S. in 1978) and today, as that paint flakes or becomes dust, it may be ingested or inhaled.

Children are more at risk for lead exposure than adults because they have smaller bodies that are developing and their behavior puts them at an increased risk. Children are more likely to pick up the sweet tasting lead flakes and eat them, or crawl on dusty floors and then lick their fingers. Because of this, children should have their blood levels tested at 1 or 2 years of age. Home handymen or weekend warriors can also cause problems when they sand materials that contain lead paint. Lead dust from sanding can be easily circulated throughout a house by natural air currents and the home's HVAC system. Once the lead dust has become airborne, it can be inhaled, and the particles that land on the tables and floor can be ingested.

Lead paint can be remediated, but contractors must take the EPA Lead Renovator and Repair training and follow the EPA protocols for lead removal. This is not only to ensure that the home is lead free but also to protect the workers as they do the removal.

Lead paint is an important issue, not only in existing buildings, but also in new buildings that use recycled materials for sustainability reasons. Salvaged wood doors and windows, in particular, may have lead paint on them, and careful attention needs to be paid when purchasing any older or salvaged materials.

Asbestos

Asbestos is a naturally occurring mineral with documented health issues from as far back as ancient Roman times. However, asbestos was widely used in building materials in the United States until the 1970s. The material is very resistant to heat and fire, making it an excellent source for insulation, and is a durable material. Asbestos can still be found in many existing buildings, in the form of siding, tiles, plumbing pipe wrap, roofing and insulation (especially vermiculite). In new buildings, the practice of sourcing salvaged material may introduce asbestos into an otherwise healthy space.

Asbestos is made up of bundles of very strong, thin, sharp threads that can float in the air for long periods of time. If these threads land on a heat source the material becomes "friable" (easily crumbled), which increases the numbers of particles in the air. When inhaled, asbestos can become trapped in the lungs. There the fibers can cause scarring and inflammation. After a period of time this may lead to asbestosis (permanent lung damage from the inflammation and scarring) and/or lung cancer or mesothelioma, a form of cancer affecting the lining of the lungs and membranes in the chest cavity.

Asbestos is still legal in the U.S. and is used in some building materials—notably cement asbestos pipes. Research has suggested that when asbestos is not friable it will pose very little risk. When there is a concern that it may become airborne, the asbestos will need to be removed by a trained professional.

Volatile Organic Compounds

Volatile Organic Compounds (VOCs) are chemicals that evaporate at room temperature from solid or liquid materials (commonly referred to as outgassing). These include such chemicals as acetone, benzene, methylene chloride, perchloroethylene and toluene. Formaldehyde is also a VOC and will be addressed in its own section. VOCs can be found in paints, cleaners, wood preservatives, solvents, vinyl floors and many more building materials. The people who live or work in the buildings where there are many sources of VOCs are at risk for many health conditions. Cleaning products, pesticides, air fresheners and personal care products are often used inside of buildings, and they all can contain VOCs. VOCs are often 2–5 times higher inside our homes than outside.[1]

VOCs may be fast decaying (they are released rapidly into the environment from the material) or slow-decaying (they tend to slowly keep releasing for a long period of time). When they are off-gassing, VOCs may be absorbed by other building materials such as drywall or carpets, and then released at a later time. This is known as the sink effect.

VOCs have been linked to headaches, eye, nose and throat irritation and damage to the kidneys, liver and central nervous system among other symptoms. Some VOCs are more toxic than others (for example, benzene is a known human carcinogen) and some people are more susceptible than others. Several states and countries, including California, regulate the levels of VOCs in consumer products. The best strategy to avoid or minimize VOCs is to only use materials or products that have low or no emissions. With the increase in green building programs across the U.S., manufacturers have responded with a wide variety of low VOC products; however, it is important to specify and verify levels of VOCs.

Formaldehyde

Formaldehyde is a VOC of specific concern. It is a colorless gas that is used in the manufacturing process of several materials commonly found in buildings, including the resin in many wood products, carpets, drapery, upholstery, varnishes and finishes and cigarettes. Formaldehyde is found in the air and its primary source of exposure is inhalation. Most of the formaldehyde that enters the lungs is broken down by the cells lining the lungs and is then exhaled. At high levels formaldehyde enters the bloodstream where it travels through our systems (including nervous and brain) and is expelled in our urine.

Formaldehyde is a very reactive molecule and as such, is an irritant to tissues such as the eyes and the respiratory tract with which it comes in contact. In 1987, a number of animal and human studies prompted the Department of Health and Human Services to label formaldehyde as a human carcinogen.[2]

Strategies to avoid formaldehyde in buildings include banning indoor cigarette smoking and creating dedicated smoking areas away from the building, limiting the use of pressed wood products and ventilating a building as much as possible for at least 10 days (open windows, for example) when new carpets or other materials containing formaldehyde are brought into the building.

Phthalates

Phthalates are a class of synthetic, semi-volatile chemicals that are used as plasticizers (a petroleum-based product) in polyvinyl chloride (PVC) products to make hard plastic more pliable. Without plasticizers plastic would be more likely to shatter from impact. Phthalates are less volatile than VOCs but are not bound to the PVC so they slowly leach out from the plastics into the air and water. They are also found in household dust in nearly every home. In buildings, they are typically found in materials such as pipes, flooring tiles, windows, carpet backing and shower curtains, and can comprise 25–50 percent of the weight of the product.[3]

Phthalates are endocrine disruptors—they interfere with the body's hormone system. The male reproductive system of young boys is most vulnerable and interference with the genital development is common.[4] A recent study also shows a strong correlation between exposure to phthalates in the womb and with childhood asthma.[5] Researchers are also looking at potential links between fetal exposure to phthalates and early onset obesity.[6]

Phthalates are found throughout our environment. They are typically inhaled or ingested, and are present in the urine of males and females of every age and ethnic group throughout the U.S., although children tend to have higher levels than adults. Phthalates are not bio accumulative (accumulating in the tissues of a living organism) and tend to pass out of the body through our urine within 24 hours of exposure. Their ubiquity in our environment, however, means that we are constantly exposed to them. A good filtration system will help remove phthalates from the air; however, they also sink in the environment and can then be found on building materials and furnishings.

There are many alternatives to petroleum-based plasticizers in building materials including bio-based plastics made of plant material such as corn, wheat, soy and rice. However, careful attention must be paid to whether chemicals or pesticides are used in the processing of these materials to ascertain whether they will be beneficial to our health and the environment. Other alternatives to petroleum-based plasticizers include bio-based alternatives derived from glucose or castor oil.

Flame-Retardants

Flame-retardant chemicals have been added to many of the furnishings, appliances and electronic items we use in our buildings. Although some controversial toxic flame-retardants are no longer on the market, there are just as many concerns about their replacements. One example is Chlorinated Tris (TDCIPP) which was used in children's pajamas in the 1970s and is now found in polyurethane foam in furniture and baby products, which in animal trials has caused cancer and DNA mutations. Fire retardants continually migrate out of materials and adhere to common dust particles that are routinely ingested or inhaled by people and pets. Again, because of children's size and higher metabolisms, they are at a high exposure risk. Also, children tend to crawl and play on the floor, put their toys or hands in their mouths and thus they ingest contaminated dust particles. Because flame-retardants can be bio accumulative, they are often found in our fat cells. As a point of interest, our brain is roughly composed of fat. Flame-retardants have been linked to cancer, endocrine disruption, low IQ, attention deficit disorder, obesity and reproductive issues.[7]

California law required flame-retardant chemicals in all furniture for decades and, being such a large market, the California law drove the entire furniture market in the U.S. This law was finally changed, and a new standard went into effect on January 1, 2015. Now, chemical free furniture can be purchased, although it is important to check whether a particular company uses chemicals or not. Even so, there is still the problem that millions of couches, pillows and other furnishings that were impregnated with flame-retardants still exist throughout our homes and buildings. Until all of these products are replaced, people will be exposed to the chemicals, which are found in everyday house dust.

Radon

The effects of radon places a person at risk of developing several different types of cancer. Radon gas is a naturally occurring, colorless and odorless decay product of radium 226, which is a decay product of uranium. In other words, uranium decays into radium, and radium decays into radon. Uranium is found in all rocks at some level, but the higher the uranium content, the higher the radon levels will be in the soil. Rocks high in uranium include shale, phosphate rock, granite and limestone. Radon molecules seep up through the air spaces in the soil beneath buildings and because of a pressure differential within the building the radon enters through small cracks in the concrete foundation, plumbing connections and sump pumps. Dirt and rock foundations allow radon to enter a building more easily. Also, some building materials (such as granite) and domestic water supplies can also expose people to radon; once the radon has released the gas, the material is safe.

Buildings are likely to have high radon levels in areas where radon is found at high levels in soils. Radon concentrations vary from region to region in the U.S. and Europe. In general, basements will have the highest concentrations of radon because there is so much contact with the soil (floor and walls). In those states where commercial or residential spaces can be found below ground, such as Maine, Massachusetts, and New York, radon exposure risk may often be much higher than in buildings where occupancy is entirely above ground.

Radon is measured in picocuries per liter (pCi/L). The EPA's action guidelines use 4 pCi/L as an annual average exposure maximum before action should be taken and estimates more than 6 million homes in the U.S. exceed this level. Radon can be tested in several ways. There is a short-term test that may not always be reliable, depending on time of year and meteorological variables such as atmospheric pressure, and wind and rain. In order to get a more accurate picture of levels over time when a short-term test shows high radon levels, a long-term test spanning three months to a year is recommended.

Radon mitigation is an important component of building design. In new buildings, porous matting or pipes under the foundation with a passive or active exhaust vent that channels radon out of the building is already mandatory in some U.S. jurisdictions. This should be a component of building design in any region of the country with moderate to high radon levels. It is much easier and cheaper to prepare for radon mitigation than to install it after the building is completed. In existing buildings, radon mitigation will be more costly. Likewise, as buildings become more airtight to achieve better energy efficiency, there is the potential for radon to enter the building and accumulate to very high levels because it can't get out. Careful attention to foundation cracks and ventilation strategies that do not depressurize the building are important design considerations.

Pollen

People who have had repeated exposure to pollen and developed immunological sensitization react to the fine powder that comes from flowering plants. Pollen floats through the air and can be inhaled or land on the body surfaces. Pollen also enters buildings through open windows and doors, and it can be tracked into a building on people's clothing and shoes, or by domestic animals. For people who have asthma or suffer from hay fever, pollen can be a trigger for an allergic reaction.

Allergic reactions to pollen can take the form of runny eyes, watery nose, coughing, sore throat and headaches. One of the best ways to control pollen is to keep windows and doors closed, have a good filtration system in the building and use a track-off system at all entries. A good track-off system can collect dirt and contaminates that would otherwise be brought into the home. A track-off system has four parts:

- Hard surfaced walkway leading to the building
- A grate-like mat that allows dirt to fall through the gaps
- A short carpet at the entry to collect fine particles and allow shoes to dry
- A hard surface floor that is easy to clean.

Dander

Dander is the name given to tiny pieces of skin that are shed by all mammals, including humans and household pets such as dogs, cats, birds and rodents. They can be microscopic in size, and they can be found floating in the air, stuck to furnishings and embedded in carpeting. The U.S. Institutes of Medicine have found sufficient evidence of a relationship between dog and cat dander and worsening of asthmatic symptoms.[8] However, most of this evidence relates to poor cleaning habits and excessive use of materials such as carpeting which serves as a sink for all forms of dander. Exposure to allergens can also contribute to upper or lower respiratory tract symptoms and lead to rashes and itchy and watering eyes.

Household animals can be a great source of comfort to people, and there is evidence to suggest that animals can help reduce symptom severity for some illnesses. However, good hygiene practices are required to minimize dander exposure. This can be done with good design that includes spaces for regular bathing of animals, air filtration devices, ensuring that surfaces can be easily cleaned and avoiding use of building materials that may serve as sinks for dander, such as carpet or fabric upholstered soft furnishings.

Pests

Rodents, cockroaches and dust mites can all trigger an allergic reaction or asthma, as we saw with pollen and dander in previous sections. Exposure to pest allergens can cause serious allergic and asthmatic reactions. Exposure to these allergens in utero or as a young child can increase the risk of developing asthma and other allergic respiratory symptoms. It is important to minimize the exposure levels of pregnant women and children. Notice the word minimize and not eliminate. This is because infants and children require some exposures in order to develop immunity. The Hygiene Hypothesis suggests that lack of exposure to parasites and infectious agents can suppress the immune system's natural development. However, these exposures cannot be too high or they can overburden the immune system. Also, pests can be carriers of disease, and their bites can lead to serious health consequences.

Strategies to eliminate pests from a building should follow the Integrated Pest Management (IPM) approach. Focus first on designing the building so cracks where a pest might enter are eliminated. Next, limit access to food, water or places to hide. Also, it is important to rely only on non-toxic management controls rather than pesticides.

Dust mites live in bedding and mattresses, and they feed off hair and skin flakes. Their body parts and fecal matter can easily become airborne float as dust, or set-tle on surfaces. When this material is inhaled it can cause an allergic reaction. Dust mites thrive best in humid environments. Encasing mattresses, pillowcases and box springs in dust mite covers best controls dust mites. Designers should also avoid using materials in a bedroom that can trap mites, such as carpets, curtains and other fabric-based products. Also, surfaces such as flooring and window treatments should be easily cleanable. The use of an air filtration system or purifier in the bedroom or even a dehumidifier can be helpful.

Bacteria

Our buildings are hosts to multiple bacteria. Researchers at the University of Oregon[9] found more than 32,964 different major groups of bacteria in one multi-purpose building. The mere presence, however, does not necessarily lead to ill health. Venti-lation strategies are extremely important to control airborne bacteria in buildings because ventilation systems can help control the spread through dilution with clean outdoor air or filtration. However, ventilation systems can become contaminated and then distribute bacteria throughout the building.

Bacteria may also be present as a result of excess moisture and dampness in the environment. Plumbing leaks, poorly flashed windows or roofs, poorly managed rainwater or groundwater and condensation on interior surfaces can all contribute to bacterial growth. In these cases, eliminating the source of the excess moisture is key to eliminating the associated bacteria.

Legionella is one well-known bacterium that grows in warm temperature water such as hot tubs, cooling towers and evaporative condensers. Exposure to the legionella bacteria is through inhalation of contaminated water, often while showering. Legionnaire's disease is a progressive pneumonia-like illness. Regular maintenance schedules for water systems, particularly in areas with immuno-compromised people who may be more susceptible is important.[10] It's important to note that Legionella requires water to be warmed and it can spread through misters used in grocery stores or on outdoor patios in hot desert climates, or any other environment where tiny water droplets can be inhaled. Some outbreaks of legionella have been linked to water-cooling towers.

Mold

Mold is present throughout our environment, both outdoors and inside. Warm, damp environments encourage microbial growth. Inside a building, mold may be present in areas where excess moisture is generated, such as bathrooms and kitchens, and anywhere that water from the outside, such as rainwater, groundwater and lawn sprinklers can penetrate into the house. The U.S. Institutes of Medicine Report of 2004[11] found sufficient evidence linking indoor exposure to mold with the following health issues: upper respiratory tract symptoms, cough and wheeze in otherwise healthy people; asthma symptoms in people with asthma; and hypersensitivity pneumonitis in individuals susceptible to that immune-mediated condition.

Eliminating the sources of moisture will eliminate the mold. Excess interior moisture can be controlled with good ventilation of areas such as bathrooms and kitchens, and monitoring plumbing connections so that they can be quickly repaired when they begin to leak. Also eliminating the use of carpeting in kitchens, bathrooms and basements where there is a higher likelihood of moisture will also aid in eliminating moisture.

Air conditioning coils can be a significant breeding ground for both mold and bacteria, which can then be circulated throughout the building through air ducts. Air with bacteria and mold spores can be blown past the coil where some are deposited on the damp coil surface. Low lighting combined with a moisture source provides an ideal environment for mold and bacteria to grow and proliferate. Ultraviolet germicidal lamps installed in air conditioning systems at the coil have been shown to reduce microbial contamination in air conditioning systems.[12]

Particulate Matter

Particulate matter (PM) refers to particles that can be inhaled. The following chart provides an overview of particulate matter size and sources (Table 6.1). Particles of most concern are those smaller than 2.5 microns (PM2.5), which are mainly the product of combustion. This may be from such things as automobiles, coal fired power plants and even indoor cooking. These small particles stay airborne longer and, when inhaled, penetrate deep into the lungs. PM2.5 has been shown to affect the respiratory and cardiovascular systems. They can also damage the cells of the respiratory tract, cause inflammation and impair the immune system. The World

TABLE 6.1 Particulate Matter Size and Sources

Source	Size and Example
Dust	About 100 microns
	EXAMPLE: Sand, cement dust, pollen
Fumes	Greater than one micron
	EXAMPLE: Products of gaseous combustion
Mist	Submicron to 20 microns
	EXAMPLE: Condensation or atomization of a liquid
Fog	Submicron to 20 microns
	Example: Visible mist
Smoke	0.05–1.0 microns
	EXAMPLE: Tobacco smoke
Smog	Less than 2 microns
	EXAMPLE: Photochemical reaction combined with water vapor

Health Organization[13] cites the health impacts as "respiratory and cardiovascular morbidity, such as aggravation of asthma, respiratory symptoms and an increase in hospital admissions; mortality from cardiovascular and respiratory diseases and from lung cancer."

Particles smaller than 0.1 microns are referred to as ultrafine particles and can enter into the bloodstream. Anything that enters the bloodstream can affect any organ including the brain. PM0.1 often come from diesel combustion engines used in ships, heavy machinery, cargo trucks and other large vehicles. Other sources of PM0.1 include hydrocarbons and metals that have become airborne through wind, traffic and regular play on or near contaminated surfaces.

Multiple studies have shown that people who live or work in buildings that are close to freeways, ports or coal-fired power plants have higher risk for cardiovascular and respiratory diseases. Designers should consider site locations for parks, bike paths and residential housing. They also need to consider the sources of air for buildings in order to ensure proper and adequate filtration systems are in place.

Common Contaminants from Equipment

Carbon Monoxide

Carbon monoxide (CO) is a colorless, odorless, tasteless and poisonous gas that is produced from incomplete combustion. In other words, if a carbon material is burned (such as wood, coal or gas) and there is not enough oxygen for the combustion process, the resulting combustion gas will include carbon monoxide. When carbon monoxide is inhaled it enters the bloodstream and binds to the hemoglobin thus reducing the availability for oxygen. At low levels, CO poisoning symptoms resembles the flu (headache, nausea, shortness of breath and dizziness). At higher levels, there can be vomiting, confusion and death. It is important to realize that

TABLE 6.2 Levels of CO Recommended by Different Organizations

Agency	Situation	Maximum CO Level	Duration
Environmental Protection Agency (EPA)	Outdoor/Ambient Air	9 ppm 35 ppm	8 hours 1 hour
Consumer Products Safety Commission/Underwriter Laboratories (UL)	Alarms for Immediate Life Threats in Residential Air	70 ppm 150 ppm 400 ppm	1–4 hours 10–50 min 4–15 min
Canadian Department of National Health & Welfare	Air in Residences	11 ppm 25 ppm	8 hours 1 hour
World Health Organization	Indoor Air	32 ppm 9 ppm 26 ppm 52 ppm 87 ppm	Max 8 hours 1 hour 30 min 15 min

Created by Amanda Hatherly

CO is often referred to as the "Silent Killer" because it is colorless and odorless, and death can occur without the person being aware that high levels exist.

The Centers for Disease Control[14] (CDC) has reported that emergency rooms treat over 15,000 people each year for carbon monoxide exposures that are non-fire related, and an average of 500 people die annually in the U.S. from non-fire related carbon monoxide exposures. Children, elders, people with compromised health and pregnant women are the most susceptible to low-level carbon monoxide poisoning. Also, people who work from home, or spend a lot of their day inside the home are at greater risk. Carbon monoxide levels are measured in parts per million (ppm). There are varying levels of CO recommended by different organizations as shown in Table 6.2.

Interior sources of carbon monoxide can include gas from fireplaces, space heaters and generators. It's important to avoid carbon monoxide poisoning by ensuring combustion gas is properly ventilated, and does not enter the home. Designers should pay attention to the location and uses of combustion producers such as hot water heaters, gas stoves and fireplaces and gas furnaces). These products should be checked annually to ensure they function without producing carbon monoxide.

Nitrogen Dioxide

Nitrogen dioxide (NO_2) is a combustion by-product of fossil fuels that negatively affects health. Like particulate matter, sources of NO_2 may derive from exterior or interior sources. The main source of external NO_2 is nearby road traffic or other combustion-based business such shipping ports or factories. Within the interior NO_2 typically comes from poorly vented appliances such as furnaces and water heaters. Attached garages and fireplaces are two other potential sources. Gas stoves and ovens, as mentioned earlier, may have no ventilation associated with them, or they may have ineffective ventilation (clogged with grease from years of cooking). Cooking is often seen as the largest contributor to indoor NO2 levels in many older and low-income homes. Other sources of NO2 within the interior environment are candles, mosquito coils and incense.

Nitrogen dioxide irritates our eyes, nose and throat and can cause inflammation of the airways. It is associated with increased respiratory infections in young children and exacerbation of asthma.[15] To eliminate the effects of NO2 it's important to ensure proper venting and exhausting of internal combustion contaminants. Range hoods should be properly specified and designers need to be aware of the range hood's capture efficiency, which varies substantially.[16] Range hoods should also be designed so that they can be cleaned regularly and tested to ensure they function appropriately effectively. Also designers should be aware of the different services and business operations within the surrounding geography. Areas close to factories, freeways or shipping should have a tighter sealed building to minimize exterior sources of NO2 from entering the building.

Ozone

Ozone is a highly reactive and unstable gas. It irritates the respiratory tract (nose, throat and airways), and the lungs, and high concentrations of ozone can irritate the eyes. Inside buildings, ozone is produced by photocopiers, laser printers and in spaces with a lot of electronic equipment. Computer servers, photocopiers and printers should be located in a dedicated space away from the primary work area, and in a well-ventilated space with a direct exhaust.

Conclusion

There are several specific contaminants found in the built environment. These contaminants are often inhaled or ingested. Many of these contaminates can remain in a building for years because they get stored in various "sinks" such as carpeting. The degree of "tightness" of a building can help conserve energy and prevent exterior sources of contaminants from entering a building, but a tight building will also prevent interior contaminates from getting out. This can cause an unhealthy mixture of different contaminants. Appropriate ventilation is an excellent strategy to keep external contaminants out while pulling interior contaminants out of the building.

The best strategy to reduce exposure to contaminants is to locate housing away from industrial areas, office workers away from high polluting office equipment and to consult with landscape architects to reduce high pollenating vegetation within areas where children, the elderly and the immune-compromised inhabit. It's also important for interior designers to be aware of where products are produced and from what those products are made. We should be thinking about keeping sources of VOCs out of the built environment all together, and ensuring that equipment such as a range hoods have optimal performance.

When it comes to environmental contaminants, prevention is the most cost effective and health enhancing practice. Prevention is tied to proactive environmental policy, a good site analysis, awareness of what goes into building products and specifying the most efficient, effective and environmentally sustaining products possible.

Notes

1 Lance A. Wallace, "The Total Exposure Assessment Methodology (TEAM) Study: Summary and Analysis: Volume I," *Office of Research and Development US Environmental Protection Agency* 600 (September 1987): 6–87.
2 National Institute for Occupational Safety and Health, "Formaldehyde: Evidence of Carcinogenicity," Centers for Disease Control, www.cdc.gov/niosh/docs/81-111/.
3 Thad Godish, *Indoor Environmental Quality* (Boca Raton, FL: CRC Press, November 2, 2007).
4 Carl-Gustaf Bornehag, Fredrik Carlstedt, Bo A. G. Jönsson, Christian H. Lindh, Tina K. Jensen, Anna Bodin, Carin Jonsson, Staffan Janson, and Shanna H. Swan, "Prenatal Phthalate Exposures and Anogenital Distance in Swedish Boys," *Environmental Health Perspectives* 123, no. 1 (2015): 101.
5 Robin M. Whyatt, Matthew S. Perzanowski, Allan C. Just, Andrew G. Rundle, Kathleen M. Donohue, Antonia M. Calafat, Lori A. Hoepner, Frederica P. Perera, and Rachel L. Miller, "Asthma in Inner-City Children at 5–11 Years of Age and Prenatal Exposure to Phthalates: The Columbia Center for Children's Environmental Health Cohort," *Environmental Health Perspectives* 122, no. 10 (2014): 1141.
6 Shin Hye Kim and Mi Jung Park, "Phthalate Exposure and Childhood Obesity," *Annals of Pediatric Endocrinology & Metabolism* 19, no. 2 (2014): 69–75.
7 Brenda Eskenazi, Jonathan Chevrier, Stephen A. Rauch, Katherine Kogut, Kim G. Harley, Caroline Johnson, Celina Trujillo, Andreas Sjödin, and Asa Bradman, "In Utero and Childhood Polybrominated Diphenyl Ether (PBDE) Exposures and Neurodevelopment in the CHAMACOS Study," *Environmental Health Perspectives* 121, no. 2 (February 2015): 257–262.
8 Institute of Medicine, *Clearing the Air: Asthma and Indoor Air Exposures* (Washington, DC: National Academy Press, 2000).
9 Steven W. Kembel, James F. Meadow, Timothy K. O'Connor, Gwynne Mhuireach, Dale Northcutt, Jeff Kline, Maxwell Moriyama, G. Z. Brown, Brendan J. M. Bohannan, and Jessica L. Green, "Architectural Design Drives the Biogeography of Indoor Bacterial Communities," *PLoS One* 9, no. 1 (2014): 1–10.
10 James F. Meadow, Adam E. Altrichter, Steven W. Kembel, J. Kline, Gwynne A. Mhuireach, Moriyama Maxwell, Dale Northcutt, Timothy K. O'Connor, Ann M. Womack, G. Z. Brown, Jessica L. Green, and Brendan J. M. Bohannan, "Indoor Airborne Bacterial Communities Are Influenced by Ventilation, Occupancy, and Outdoor Air Source," *Indoor Air* 24, no. 1 (2014): 41–48.
11 Committee on Damp Indoor Spaces and Health; Board on Health Promotion and Disease Prevention; Institute of Medicine, *Damp Indoor Spaces and Health* (Washington, DC: National Academies Press, 2004).
12 Dick Menzies, Julia Popa, James A. Hanley, Thomas Rand, and Donald K. Milton, "Effect of Ultraviolet Germicidal Lights Installed in Office Ventilation Systems on Workers' Health and Well-being: Double-Blind Multiple Crossover Trial," *The Lancet* 362, no. 9398 (November 2003): 1785–1791.
13 World Health Organization, *Health Effects of Particulate Matter: Policy Implications for Countries in Eastern Europe, Caucasus and Central Asia* (Copenhagen, Denmark: World Health Organization, 2013).
14 Center for Disease Control and Prevention, "Carbon Monoxide Exposures: United States, 2000–2009," *Morbidity and Mortality Weekly* 60, no. 30 (August 2011): 1014–1017.
15 Institute of Medicine, *Clearing the Air*, 2000.
16 Nate Seltenrich, "Take Care in the Kitchen: Avoiding Cooking-Related Pollutants," *Environmental Health Perspectives* 122, no. 6 (2014): A154.

7

GREEN DESIGN AND HEALTH

Sherry Ahrentzen, Elif Tural, and James Erickson

Introduction

With growing research and building industry initiatives such as USGBC (United States Green Building Council), BREEAM (the UK's Building Research Establishment Environmental Assessment Method) and Australia's Green Star program, the notion that "green is good" has made its way into public awareness. Surveys show increasing interest in green design and construction among the general public, as well as those in the design, construction and real estate development industries.[1] The green building movement is becoming more prominent in many countries, and green building practices are increasingly embedded in building, financing and policy regulations. Many corporations, public agencies, non-profits, hospitals and academic institutions are stipulating green in their building guidelines and real estate portfolios.[2]

ABBREVIATIONS IN THIS CHAPTER

ASHRAE: American Society of Heating, Refrigerating and Air-conditioning Engineers
EGC: Enterprise Community Partners' Green Communities Certification
HR Standards: Health-related Standards (includes NHHS and WELL-MF)
IAQ: Indoor Air Quality
LEED: LEED for Homes Design and Construction
NHHS: National Healthy Housing Standard
VOCs: Volatile Organic Compounds
WELL-MF: WELL Multifamily Residential Pilot Addendum
WHO: World Health Organization

To many, "green design" and "health" may seem symbiotic, if not synonymous. But recent research by environmental health scientists[3] suggests that while the two sometimes correspond, they also sometimes conflict. For example, initial green building efforts targeted extremely tight building envelopes with minimal indoor-outdoor air exchange to maximize energy efficiency. An unintended consequence was intensified exposures to indoor toxins that resulted in respiratory and other detrimental health outcomes. Probing the health benefits and shortcomings of green building practices continues today even though some of these green practices have changed (such as adjustments in indoor-outdoor air exchange). As designers, what confidence can we have that when we follow green building practices we not only "do no harm" (as in the Hippocratic oath) but also that we advance and foster the health and wellness of the building occupants?

In 2006, the National Center for Healthy Housing produced a report that compared five green building certification programs with seven healthy homes principles.[4] Our analysis here updates and expands upon that earlier work. Since "green design" is an umbrella term for a wide range of practices, in this chapter we focus on green design as encapsulated in two green certification programs used in the U.S. that cover residential structures and settings: USGBC's *LEED for Homes* and Enterprise Community Partners' *Green Communities Criteria*. Since it would be overwhelming to cover all building types in a single chapter, we have chosen to target residential structures since those are settings where people spend much of their lives, and also where the most vulnerable populations—young children, older adults and the infirm—spend most of their time.[5] Some researchers believe that shifts in ambient conditions due to climate change will lead to people spending even more time indoors.[6]

This chapter first provides a brief overview of leading health-related impacts of indoor building factors. Many health concerns pertaining to the residential environment have been captured in two national health-related building standards: WELL and National Healthy Housing Standard (NHHS). Following our description of these, we analyze how LEED for Homes and Green Communities guidelines reflect, neglect or even potentially contradict these health-related building standards—and ways in which designers need to responsibly apply green guidelines as to ensure, or at least not compromise, occupant health. The chapter ends with some lessons learned from the analysis.

Health Concerns at Home

Research indicates that indoor residential factors may be associated with numerous health conditions: stress and depression (due to housing quality, household density and crowding, noise); cardiovascular disease (from VOCs, sedentary behavior); lung cancer (from radon); neurological disorders (from lead); chronic respiratory diseases including asthma (from pests, animal dander, environmental tobacco smoke, humidity, heat, dust mites); infectious diseases (poor sanitation and hygienic conditions); mortality (excessive heat or cold); injuries such as falls or scalds (from hazards, fixtures); and obesity and its related illnesses such as diabetes (from environmental factors that support sedentary behavior).[7]

While building and housing codes address some of the egregious building factors that can threaten health and safety—such as evenness of stair treads or lead-free paint—existing codes often do not include comprehensive health responses, nor address more chronic health conditions such as maintaining dry environments to reduce mold and mildew that exacerbate asthma.

There are several reviews that document and describe the research evidence on how environmental, physical and spatial factors of residences impact occupant health.[8] As a boon to designers, two important initiatives have used this research evidence to craft residential building and design standards related to health. Developed by the National Center for Healthy Housing (NCHH) and the American Public Health Association (APHA), the *National Healthy Housing Standard* (herein referred to as "NHHS") is an evidence-based tool and standard of care to improve housing conditions related to occupant health. It targets housing undergoing renovation. This U.S. standard is a modified version of one produced by the UK government, *Housing Health and Safety Rating System.*[9] NHHS addresses: duties of owners and occupants; structures, facilities, plumbing and space requirements; safety and personal security; lighting and electrical systems; thermal comfort, ventilation and energy efficiency; moisture control, solid waste and pest management; and chemical and radiological agents.

While the NHHS primarily stipulates *minimum* performance standards, it also includes provisions called "*stretch*" that could be added to further enhance the health and safety of the home's occupants, recognizing that these may be difficult to achieve for some properties due to cost or feasibility. Written in code language to ease its adoption, the NHHS is seen as a bridge between health codes and building codes by putting modern public health information into housing code language.[10]

The second health-related building standard is that developed by the International WELL Building Institute.[11] The initial WELL standard targeted commercial and institutional buildings, but has been followed by a pilot version (as of this date) for multifamily residential buildings (herein referred to as WELL-MF).[12] Each feature is ascribed to one or more human body systems that are intended to benefit from its implementation: cardiovascular, digestive, endocrine, immune, integumentary, muscular, nervous, reproductive, respiratory, skeletal and urinary. According to its document, WELL Building Standard was developed by integrating scientific and medical research and reviewing existing literature on environmental health, behavioral factors, health outcomes and demographic risk factors.

The Standard is organized into seven categories of wellness: Air, Water, Nourishment, Light, Fitness, Comfort and Mind. Similar to the two-tier system of NHHS, WELL features are designated as either *Preconditions* (i.e., they must be met), or *Optimizations* (i.e., encouraged to gain higher levels of certification). Unlike NHHS, WELL targets both new construction and renovation.

While there is some overlap between the two standards, each addresses unique health-related building concerns, or addresses a particular health concern in more

depth than the other standard does. As a result, our analyses of the two green certification programs were based on their correspondence with occupant health-based
standards in both NHHS and WELL-MF.

Do Green Building Programs Reflect Health-Related Building Standards?

When comparing the health-related building recommendations in NHHS and
WELL-MF to green design certification programs, we focused the latter on *LEED
Reference Guide for Homes Design and Construction* version 4[13] and *Enterprise Green
Communities 2015 Criteria and Certification*.[14] (Hereafter, these are referred to as
LEED and EGC, respectively.)

Our process involved identifying those WELL-MF Features and NHHS Requirements Provisions (henceforth, these are collectively referred to as *Health-Related
Standards,* or *HR Standards*) that represented one of six categories:

(1) Chemical Contaminants in IAQ
(2) Biological Contaminants in IAQ
(3) Ventilation
(4) Thermal Conditions
(5) Water
(6) Lighting

After reviewing HR Standards for each category, we examined the guidelines in
LEED and EGC to gauge correspondence. We assembled this coded information
in an extensive multi-matrix format to use as the foundation for our analyses and
interpretation, which follows below.

Chemical Contaminants in IAQ

Indoor air pollution poses many challenges to design professionals. It has immediate health effects, such as irritation of the eyes, nose and throat, headaches, dizziness
and fatigue, and long-term outcomes, including asthma, allergies, other respiratory
conditions, cardiovascular diseases and cancer.[15] Major sources of chemical pollutants in indoor air include: gases and particles from fuel-burning combustion
appliances (such as ranges, ovens, fireplaces), tobacco products, VOCs released from
building materials and furnishings, deteriorated asbestos- or lead-containing building materials, household cleaning and maintenance products and outdoor sources
brought indoors, such as pesticides, radon and outdoor air pollution.[16] The amount,
duration of exposure and hazardousness of contaminants released into the air affect
the degree and scope of health impacts.

The U.S. Environmental Protection Agency (EPA) sets exposure limits for some
chemical pollutants but does not regulate indoor air quality.[17] While it maintains a
list of potentially toxic substances, there are no testing requirements or regulations

for most of the chemicals used extensively by the building industry, such as phthalates used in vinyl products and PBDEs used as flame-retardants.[18] The World Health Organization (WHO) and the American Society of Heating, Refrigerating and Air-Conditioning Engineers (ASHRAE) provide guidelines and standards for air quality and ventilation.[19] Certain states, such as California and New Jersey, set their own more restrictive, indoor air quality standards, but with no, or limited, correspondence to residential environments.[20] The extent to which these exposure standards are adopted in the HR Standards and green design certification programs varies considerably.

The most effective way to improve IAQ is pollutant source removal and control.[21] Another viable technique is increasing ventilation and filtering particles and volatile pollutants. Since ventilation is examined in a later section, this section primarily focuses on source control and air quality monitoring.

How LEED Measures Up

Several indoor air quality prerequisites or credits regarding chemicals are either insufficient to meet HR Standards, or sometimes conflict with them. For example, the energy and atmosphere credits related to envelope insulation emphasize R-values to conserve energy, rather than the potential toxins that can emit from insulation materials to indoors. Both WELL-MF and LEED allow and award points for use of polystyrene insulation and polyurethane foam insulation despite the concerns about the use of HBCD and other flame-retardants found in these building materials.[22] Another potential adverse health effect relates to the materials and resources credit on environmentally preferable products—with no requirement for testing potential toxic emissions from reclaimed, post- and pre-consumer recycled and recyclable products.

Since WELL-MF's VOC reduction standards are partially based on a LEED guideline (i.e., EQ Credit: Low-emitting materials), the LEED credits essentially echo WELL-MF. The main difference is that satisfying these measures are *required* in WELL, but *optional* in LEED. Use of PVC and plasticizers including phthalates, and other chemicals, such as BPAs and PFOAs, found in building materials are allowed in LEED buildings, and no credits are provided for avoiding them.

On the positive side, an innovation credit that awards a point for selecting products with manufacturer disclosed chemical ingredients or third-party verified harmful substance reduction—such as GreenScreen v.1.2 Benchmark—is an indication that LEED recognizes the need to incorporate this issue to its standards. Additionally, LEED now offers a pilot credit for prevention of pollution from construction equipment and vehicles.

With respect to air quality, LEED does not require air quality testing after occupancy. Testing for smaller particulate matter (PM) and VOCs (including formaldehyde) is optional, and testing is conducted pre-occupancy. While LEED's outdoor smoking ban is in sync with WELL-MF requirements, it only requires an indoor smoking ban in common areas of multifamily projects, with an optional credit to prohibit smoking in the entire building.

Along with smoking and secondhand smoke, radon is one of the leading causes of lung cancer and there is direct evidence linking residential radon exposure and lung cancer.[23] LEED has a radon-resistant construction prerequisite for buildings in high-risk zones (EPA radon zone 1) and requirement for an active ventilation system for renovation buildings if radon levels are greater than 4pCi/L. However, EPA recommends radon level testing regardless of location.[24] While LEED-HDC has an innovation credit awarded in moderate-risk areas for radon-resistant construction, the current standard fails to ensure radon safety in all residential construction.

How EGC Measures Up

Similar to LEED, EGC lacks requirements for air quality testing and mitigation after occupancy. While EGC's requirements for no or low VOC materials support indoor air quality and asthmagen-free materials credit are a step ahead of LEED, EGC's optional smoking ban falls short to minimize tobacco smoke exposure of occupants. While EGC has mandatory requirements for combustion equipment venting and requires full compliance with ASHRAE 62.2 ventilation standards, it does not address construction pollution management issues. EGC also falls short in addressing asbestos and methamphetamine testing and abatement requirements of NHHS. Lastly, EGC's handling of radon is similar to LEED. Except for rehabilitation projects, there is no requirement for radon testing at the lowest occupied level pre- or post-occupancy.

Summary

In general, neither green design program seems to ensure occupant health by comprehensively eliminating, controlling, monitoring and mitigating toxic chemicals indoors to the extent advanced by the HR Standards. While EGC has stricter requirements pertaining to VOCs, LEED's innovation credit for material ingredients may suggest a positive change in approach to occupant health. Nonetheless, designers and builders need to take a proactive role for prioritizing health from indoor toxic substances discussed later in the Conclusions.

Biological Contaminants in IAQ

Biological pollutants come from living organisms dwelling in and around the home. Common sources of biological air contaminants include, but are not limited to: animal dander; fungi and molds; some infectious agents (e.g., Legionella); pollen from surrounding plants; mites, cockroaches and other common indoor pests and their excretions. Contaminants can find their way into the home through a variety of means: air infiltration and filtration systems; transmission by shoe soles of humans, paws of pets and the like; dampness in basements and bathrooms; and rodents and other pests.[25]

While some of these pollutants are found in every home in varying concentration levels, many can be controlled through good house cleaning, proper maintenance of the home including the ventilation system and managing indoor moisture levels. Decisions made during the design process can help shape this control, such as the choice of antimicrobial surfaces in kitchens and bathrooms, moisture resistant finishes and effective ventilation and filtration. Since it is not practical to create home designs that eliminate *all* biological contaminates, design strategies that facilitate ongoing care and maintenance are ideal to reducing time and effort expended by occupants in the care of their home. Too, the designer's choice of materials and ventilation systems, and the design of entry spaces, for example, can assist in preventing biologically-based pollutants through active filtration systems and ventilation.

How Do LEED and EGC Measure Up?

Generally, LEED and EGC do not directly address biological IAQ issues; and when they do, guidelines are limited to initial design strategies, not maintenance (an issue addressed in the Conclusions). For example, what is framed as a health concern in the WELL standard for preventing mold growth and the aerosolization of microbes, LEED presents as a comfort issue by citing ASHRAE 62.2 requirements for indoor relative humidity control.

EGC provides more extensive measures and targets a wider range of home locations in preventing allergens and biological contaminants than LEED. LEED specifies measures for minimizing mold growth and aerosolization of microbes through ventilation/exhaust and filters. EGC, however, identifies measures to reduce mold growth in kitchens, bathrooms, water heaters and laundries through materials and ventilation; recommends vapor retardants; and requires Integrated Pest Management (IPM). However, neither green program addresses the general need for designing homes that facilitate easy cleaning to the extent that WELL-MF, and to a lesser degree NHHS, prescribe. LEED presents an optional credit for either permanent walk-off mats or a shoe removal and storage area near the main entrance. EGC does not address either.

Summary

Guidelines for ongoing maintenance and home upkeep that reduce opportunities for biological contaminants to fester are notably lacking in both green certification programs, although extensively maintained by the HR Standards. Relatively simple design solutions such as the choice of materials that are easy to clean and antimicrobial surfaces would require minimal effort to implement in these green programs.

For example, designing homes to minimize or eliminate these various IAQ containments may seem daunting, but the developer, architect and builder of the High Point Breathe-Easy Homes in Seattle, Washington (Figure 7.1), made deliberate

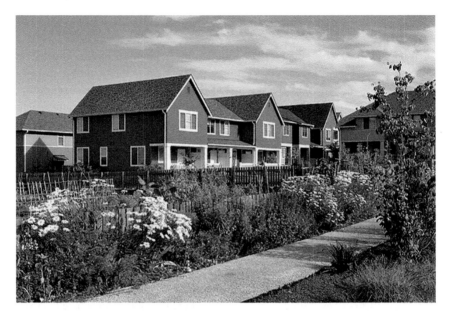

FIGURE 7.1   High Point, Seattle, Washington

Source: Photo courtesy of Mithun

efforts to address respiratory ailments through IAQ-focused features and design, all the while building to EGC standards.

Among the features were: insulated windows and foundation; an advanced air filtration system with filtered fresh air intake ports in all living spaces; positive whole house ventilation systems that removed stale air and filtered incoming air and reduced moisture; low/no off-gas trim and mill work to reduce urea formaldehyde bonding agents; HEPA filter vacuums; walk-off doormats to reduce dirt in the homes; window blinds instead of curtains to reduce dust; and special attention to protect building materials from moisture during construction (Figure 7.2).[26]

A longitudinal study of the health impacts showed greatly reduced asthma triggers and symptoms. Asthmatic children had 63 percent more symptom-free days than in their previous homes and showed dramatic improvements in lung function. Health improvements resulted in a 66 percent reduction in the need for urgent medical care.[27]

Ventilation

Both natural and mechanical ventilation systems are intended to provide fresh outdoor air to the building's occupants for achieving acceptable indoor air quality standards.[28] Proper ventilation is necessary to purge indoor environments of chemical, biological and particulate pollutants that can cause health problems and also affect an occupant's thermal comfort.

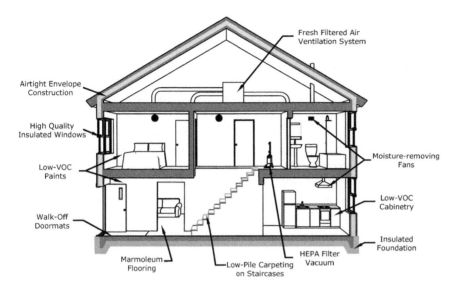

Fresh Filtered Air
Ventilation System

Airtight Envelope
Construction

High Quality
Insulated Windows

Low-VOC
Paints

Walk-Off
Doormats

Moisture-removing
Fans

Low-VOC
Cabinetry

Insulated
Foundation

Marmoleum
Flooring

Low-Pile Carpeting
on Staircases

HEPA Filter
Vacuum

FIGURE 7.2 Specific Health-Related Building Features in High Point Breathe-Easy
Homes, Seattle, Washington

Source: Diagram by James Erickson, adapted from one by Steve Barham, Neighborhood House, in
Takaro et al. 2011

Cases of Sick Building Syndrome—a term used to describe indoor environmental conditions that cause occupants acute health and comfort issues, such as fatigue, nausea, headaches and concentration difficulties[29]—are often traced to inadequate ventilation issues such as a poorly designed or maintained ventilation systems, or low airflow rates.[30] Effects from long-term exposure to poorly ventilated spaces can manifest years later as respiratory conditions, cardiovascular diseases and cancer.[31] Deaths stemming from poor ventilation are not uncommon, particularly related to carbon monoxide poisoning in homes.[32]

Many HVAC systems recirculate indoor air to minimize energy use in conditioning air to desired temperatures. However, without adequate levels of added fresh outdoor air, residential construction of tight air barriers that limit air leakage though the home's envelope can trap pollutants indoors, exposing occupants to concentrated levels of chemicals, allergens and particulate matter. The known dangers of inadequate ventilation have resulted in recommended minimum airflow rates for indoor ventilation.[33]

Ensuring a constant flow of fresh air significantly improves indoor air quality, but often times simply conditioning incoming fresh air may be inadequate to ensure that target indoor air quality standards are met. Factors such as where the fresh air intake is located, changes in outdoor air quality, changes between seasons and differing occupant sensitivity—all may require additional measures for controlling indoor air pollutants such as added air filtration and entry vestibules to help control many pollutants that contribute to chronic health issues.

How Do LEED-HDC and EGC Measure Up?

While LEED's and EGC's natural ventilation guidelines are primarily intended as a means to reduce energy, they collaterally improve indoor air circulation and reduce dependence on mechanical systems by allowing occupants to take advantage of pleasing outdoor temperatures. Yet, beyond EGC's recommended placement of windows for maximizing cross-ventilation and LEED's minimum flow rate requirements, they do not achieve the high bar for occupant health set by WELL-MF that includes monitoring of outdoor air quality and window operation management (e.g., additional filtration abilities and monitoring equipment).

And while both WELL-MF and NHHS address ongoing maintenance and operation of installed mechanical ventilation systems, attention to maintenance issues is lacking in LEED and EGC. Proper maintenance and operation are crucial to ensuring a home's ventilation system does not become a source of chronic health issues and deteriorating indoor environmental quality.[34] Although all set compliance requirements to ASHRAE 62.1 or 62.2, the HR Standards emphasize that ventilation is not simply an initial installation decision but one that needs regular attention to ensure a healthy indoor environment.

Thermal Conditions

Individuals in good general health generally adapt to changes in ambient temperature within certain limits. When temperatures push the upper end of those limits or occur with high humidity or strenuous activity, the body's thermoregulatory system can be overwhelmed, resulting in moderate to severe illnesses, even death (e.g. during extended heat waves).

ASHRAE's *Thermal Environmental Conditions for Human Occupancy* Standard 55 is often referenced for ensuring optimal thermal comfort conditions for occupants. Its graphic comfort zone method in establishing an acceptable range of operative temperature and humidity takes into account clothing insulation, metabolic rate, radiant temperature, air temperature and speed and relative humidity. Accordingly, the indoor summer comfort temperatures range from 74–83°F (23–28°C) and for winter, from 67–79°F (19–26°C), depending on the relative humidity. It separately defines acceptable temperature ranges for naturally ventilated spaces as a function of outdoor temperatures spanning 50–93°F (10–34°C).[35]

While most manufacturers, builders, engineers, architects and code officials adhere to these standards, it is worthwhile to note that the research upon which the formulas and metrics are based pertain to sedentary or near sedentary physical activity levels typical of office work. While ASHRAE claims it is acceptable to use these standards to determine appropriate environmental conditions for single family and multifamily residential construction,[36] it also states that it does not apply to sleeping or bed rest, and that the data does not incorporate significant information regarding children, the disabled, older adults or the infirm. Yet, research shows striking differences of how temperatures differentially affect health between younger and older populations.[37] As people age, their ability to cope with external environmental stressors decreases because of a number of physiological and social factors: interactions between medications and the body's heat-compensation mechanisms, isolation and decreased organ function, particularly the peripheral nervous systems which is instrumental in thermoregulation.[38]

Another indoor thermal condition affecting health is relative humidity (RH). High RH may induce conditions that foster mold, allergens and dust mites (see earlier section on Biological Pollutants). Yet, in quite arid climates such as the American Southwest, very low levels are also of concern since low RH can result in dry noses and throats that make people more susceptible to upper respiratory illnesses. Low RH levels can also facilitate skin dryness and irritation.[39]

How LEED and EGC Measure Up

Our analysis shows that EGC does not go beyond the basic required HR Standards. There are no criteria in the EGC guidelines that recommend WELL optimization or NHHS stretch standards such as programmable thermostats, real-time displays of temperature and humidity or HVAC systems that automatically maintain RH below 60 percent. In LEED, thermal comfort is addressed in ventilation and HVAC guidelines although the priority is on energy efficiency and ventilation requirements. There is a credit for zoning and room-by-room controls to improve thermal comfort, but these are not mandatory and are given minimal credit.

Summary

The green certification guidelines address most of the required HR Standards related to thermal conditions but do not go beyond these to optimal or stretch ones. Yet, these latter Standards may be of particular relevance for achieving optimal thermal conditions for the health of vulnerable occupants (such as frail older adults) in addition to concerns about the impacts that climate change will create on the thermal conditions of our residential structures.[40]

Water

The Safe Drinking Water Act (SDWA) of 1974 authorized the U.S. Environmental Protection Agency (EPA) to set and enforce health standards for contaminants in the drinking water supply and protect surface water quality. Water is tested and deemed "clean" according to the existing SDWA quality standards at the water filtration plant, but SDWA does not regulate "mixtures of pollutants in drinking water."[41] In the light of disease outbreaks, drought-related water restrictions, recent water contamination problems and the nations' aging water infrastructure, even the EPA has recognized that drinking water quality cannot be taken for granted anymore.[42] Health professionals call for water quality testing for turbidity, microorganisms, metals, organic pollutants, agricultural contaminants and public water additives. Another concern is that the EPA only regulates public water systems, not private wells that provide water for about 15 percent of Americans.[43]

How LEED Measures Up

With a focus on water efficiency, LEED relies on EPA water quality standards and has no prerequisites or credits for drinking water quality assurance. Additionally, the requirement to develop an Integrated Pest Management (IPM) to guide residents' pesticide use may not be sufficient to prevent the risk of local (well) water contamination. A potential health conflict lies in LEED's failure to prohibit, or at least, discourage use of artificial turf which potentially has adverse health effects.[44]

How EGC Measures Up

EGC addresses water as a natural resource, rather than a human health resource. EGC targets water conservation with efficient plumbing systems, water harvesting and graywater use for landscaping, minimizing leaks and water metering, but fails to set standards for contaminant levels and requirements for water quality testing. Similar to LEED, EGC does not address private water supplies, nor does it require verification that minimum standards highlighted in NHSS or WELL are met.

Summary

While LEED and EGC have potential positive impacts on surface and underground water quality protection, neither green standard tests water for chemical or biological contaminants, or requires safe limits for contaminants. To support occupant health, water quality assurance is needed from continuous onsite testing and treatment when required.

Lighting

Light impacts health and functioning by enabling vision and task performance. Light's non-visual influences on the human body include melatonin suppression, elevated cortisol production, increased core temperature and resetting the internal circadian body clock[45]—which consequently affects mood, perception and direct absorption of critical chemical reactions in the body such as Vitamin D.[46] Lighting systems are designed in compliance with lighting codes and guidelines to meet illuminance recommendations for user task performance and energy consumption limits. While the research on health effects of artificial light, including effect of the blue-light component of LEDs on the retina, is not yet conclusive,[47] studies show that adequate exposure to light, particularly daylighting, is critical for health and well-being.[48]

How Do LEED and EGC Measure Up?

Even though LEED has traditionally promoted daylighting, lighting design credits prioritize energy efficiency through solar design and energy efficient luminaires, with no correspondence to the daylight access requirements of WELL-MF and NHSS. While solar glare avoidance is addressed to some extent, electric light glare control—a precondition of WELL-MF—is missing from LEED. Most importantly, the current LEED does not include prerequisites or credits to encourage lighting design that takes circadian and sleep rhythms into consideration.

Similarly, EGC emphasizes energy efficiency and passive solar design. While the importance of daylighting is considered for mental health and active living impacts in the context of stairways and outdoors, EGC's primary concern seems to be on high-efficacy light fixtures with no mandatory daylight access and glare control requirements. Like LEED, this green standard relies on IES (Illuminating Engineering Society) guidelines and health and safety codes for lighting quantity although the need for "improved lighting" is mentioned for fall prevention. There is no correspondence to WELL-MF's sophisticated circadian lighting design guidelines.

Summary

In conclusion, both green certification programs prioritize energy efficiency over occupant health and well-being with respect to access to natural light, circadian and sleep concerns and glare. Neither program addresses light quality, i.e., light color quality (color rendering index, or CRI) and surface reflectance values (LRV). Surprisingly, however, LEED O+M (Operations and Maintenance): MF guidelines include credits for daylight access in living spaces and lighting quality (CRI and LRV values). However, since residential architects and designers usually work with LEED's Design and Construction (D+C) rating system, elimination of these credits from LEED D+C likely results in not addressing such health-related criteria in initial designs.

Conclusions

One lesson to draw from this analysis is that green building addresses a certain segment of health-related occupancy concerns, but it is far from being comprehensive. And in a few instances, green design and construction guidelines may even complicate occupant health. For those architects and builders who want to design residences that are both green and healthy, at this time it is prudent to follow the guidelines of multiple certification systems.

While design and construction guidance for addressing occupant health is advancing with the development of these two occupant health-based standards—WELL-MF and NHHS—they, like the green certification programs, will likely continually evolve. Ironically, two health-related issues we did not address in this chapter—Active Design and Inclusive (or Universal) Design—are more prominent in the green certification programs than in these two HR Standards. Growing research demonstrates environmental factors that enhance mobility and accessibility in the home that go beyond current governmental mandates (such as the Fair Housing Amendments Acts that governs accessibility issues in multifamily housing construction in the U.S.) are important in affirming health as well as reducing health care costs, particularly for older adults.[49]

Lastly, it is critical to point out that many health-related guidelines are contained in the LEED Operations and Maintenance (O+M) programs. Our analysis here was intended to cover green guidelines that designers are more likely to use and incorporate in their design work, and not necessarily the O+M material. Nonetheless, designers can make it easy or challenging for maintaining and operating a healthy home by the materials they select, the components they include and the spaces they design. While we pointed to some of these instances in our analyses, there are many more opportunities for this to occur. The integrated design process—which is advanced as a major sustainable building principle by most green building certification programs for institutional and commercial buildings—may need to incorporate facility management's critical role in multifamily housing, to ensure that "sustaining high performance" not only reflects energy efficiency but occupant health as well.

Notes

1 McGraw Hill Construction, *The Drive Towards Healthier Buildings* (New York: McGraw Hill Construction, 2014), www.aia.org/aiaucmp/groups/aia/documents/pdf/aiab104164.pdf.
2 Ibid.
3 Joseph G. Allen, Piers MacNaughton, Jose Guillermo Cedeno Laurent, Skye S. Flanigan, Erika Sita Eitland, and John D. Spengler, "Green Buildings and Health," *Current Environmental Health Reports* 2 (2015): 250; John Wargo, *LEED Certification: Where Energy Efficiency Collides With Human Health* (North Haven, CT: Environmental and Human Health Inc., 2010), www.ehhi.org/reports/leed/LEED_report_0510.pdf.
4 National Center for Healthy Housing, *Comparing Green Building Guidelines and Healthy Homes Principles: A Preliminary Investigation* (Columbia, MD: National Center for Healthy Housing, 2006), www.nchh.org/portals/0/contents/green_analysis.pdf.
5 Michael A. Berry, "Indoor Air Quality: Assessing Health Impacts and Risks," *Toxicology and Industrial Health* 7, no. 5–6 (1991): 179; Elaine A. Cohen-Hubal, Linda S. Sheldon, Janet M. Burke, Thomas R. McCurdy, Maurice R. Berry, Marc L. Rigas, Valerie G. Zartarian, and Natalie C. G. Freema, "Children's Exposure Assessment: A Review of Factors Influencing Children's Exposure, and the Data Available to Characterize and Assess That Exposure," *Environmental Health Exposure* 108, no. 6 (2000): 475; EPA, *Descriptive Statistics Tables From a Detailed Analysis of the National Human Activity Pattern Survey (NHAPS) Data* (Washington, DC: USEPA, 1996), http://publications.usa.gov/USAPubs.php?PubID=5725.
6 Philomena M. Bluyssen, *The Healthy Indoor Environment: How to Assess Occupants' Well-being in Buildings*, 1st edition (New York: Routledge, 2014); Institute of Medicine, *Climate Change, the Indoor Environment, and Health* (Washington, DC: The National Academies Press, 2011).
7 Irene Houtman, Marjolein Douwes, Tanja de Jong, Jan Michiel Meeuwsen, Mat Jongen, Frank Brekelmans, Marieke Nieboer-Op de Weegh, Dick Brouwer, Seth van den Bossche, and Gerard Zwetsloot, *New Forms of Physical and Psychological Health Risks at*

Work (Brussels, Belgium: European Parliament, 2008); James Krieger, David E. Jacobs, Peter J. Ashley, Andrea Baeder, Ginger L. Chew, Dorr Dearborn, H. Patricia Hynes, J. David Miller, Rebecca Morley, Felicia Rabito, and D. C. Zeldin, "Housing Interventions and Control of Asthma-Related Indoor Biologic Agents: A Review of the Evidence," *Journal of Public Health Management and Practice* 16, no. 5 (2010): S11–S20.

8   James Krieger and Donna L. Higgins, "Housing and Health: Time Again for Public Health Action," *American Journal of Public Health* 92, no. 5 (2002): 758; Krieger et al., "Housing Interventions and Control of Asthma-Related Indoor Biologic Agents: A Review of the Evidence"; Thomas D. Matte and David E. Jacobs, "Housing and Health: Current Issues and Implications for Research and Programs," *Journal of Urban Health* 77, no. 1 (2000): 7–25; Susan C. Saegert et al., "Healthy Housing: A Structured Review of Published Evaluations of U.S. Interventions to Improve Health by Modifying Housing in the United States, 1990–2001," *American Journal of Public Health* 93, no. 9 (2003): 1471–1477; World Health Organization, "Report on the WHO Technical Meeting on Quantifying Disease From Inadequate Housing," 2006, "http://www.euro.who.int/__data/assets/pdf_file/0007/98674/EBD_Bonn_Report.pdf<http://www.euro.who.int/__data/assets/pdf_file/0007/98674/EBD_Bonn_Report.pdf" www.euro.who.int/__data/assets/pdf_file/0007/98674/EBD_Bonn_Report.pdf<http://www.euro.who.int/__data/assets/pdf_file/0007/98674/EBD_Bonn_Report.pdf

9   Department for Communities and Local Government, *Housing Health and Safety Rating System* (London: Department for Communities and Local Government, 2006), www.gov.uk/government/uploads/system/uploads/attachment_data/file/9425/150940.pdf.

10 National Center for Healthy Housing and American Public Health Association, *National Healthy Housing Standard* (Columbia, MD: National Center for Healthy Housing, 2014).

11 International WELL Building Institute, *The WELL Building Standard* (New York: International Well Building Institute, 2015), www.wellcertified.com/well.

12 International WELL Building Institute, *The WELL Multifamily Residential Pilot Addendum* (New York: International Well Building Institute, 2015), www.wellcertified.com/well.

13 USGBC, *LEED Reference Guide for Homes Design and Construction*, 2013 edition (New York: U.S. Green Building Council, 2015).

14 Enterprise Community Partners, *2015 Enterprise Green Communities* Criteria Columbia, M.D.: Enterprise Community Partners, (2015).

15 EPA, "Indoor Air Quality," www.epa.gov/indoor-air-quality-iaq; WHO, "Indoor Air Pollution: Health and Social Impacts of Household Energy," www.who.int/indoorair/health_impacts/en/.

16 EPA, "Indoor Air Quality"; OSHA, *Indoor Air Quality in Commercial and Institutional Buildings* (Washington, DC: Occupational Safety and Health Administration, 2011), www.osha.gov/Publications/3430indoor-air-quality-sm.pdf.

17 NAAQS, "U.S. National Ambient Air Quality Standards," www3.epa.gov/ttn/naaqs/criteria.html.

18 Wargo, *LEED Certification: Where Energy Efficiency Collides With Human Health*.

19 ANSI/ASHRAE, *Standard 62.2-2013 Ventilation for Acceptable Indoor Air Quality in Low-Rise Residential Buildings* (Atlanta, GA: American Society of Heating, Refrigerating, and Air-Conditioning Engineers, Inc., 2013); WHO, *Particulate Matter, Ozone, Nitrogen Dioxide and Sulfur Dioxide* (Geneva, Switzerland: World Health Organization), www.who.int/phe/health_topics/outdoorair/outdoorair_aqg/en/; WHO, *WHO Guidelines for Indoor Air Quality: Selected Pollutants* (Geneva, Switzerland: WHO Regional Office for Europe, 2010), www.euro.who.int/__data/assets/pdf_file/0009/128169/e94535.pdf; WHO, *Indoor Air Pollution: Health and Social Impacts of Household Energy*.

20 "New Jersey Indoor Air Quality Standard (N.J.A.C. 12:100-13)," 2007, www.state.nj.us/health/peosh/iaq.shtml; "Standard Method for the Testing and Evaluation of Volatile Organic Chemical Emissions From Indoor Sources Using Environmental Chambers, V. 1.1," California Department of Public Health (CDPH), 2010.

21 EPA, "Indoor Air Quality."

22 Wargo, *LEED Certification: Where Energy Efficiency Collides With Human Health*.

23 EPA, "Health Risk of Radon," www.epa.gov/radon/health-risk-radon; WHO, *WHO Handbook on Indoor Radon: A Public Health Perspective* (Geneva, Switzerland: World Health Organization), www.who.int/ionizing_radiation/env/radon/en/.

24 EPA, "Health Risk of Radon."

25 James Krieger, David E. Jacobs, Peter J. Ashley, Andrea Baeder, Ginger L. Chew, Dorr Dearborn, H. Patricia Hynes, J. David Miller, Rebecca Morley, Felicia Rabito, and D.C. Zeldin, "Housing Interventions and Control of Asthma-Related Indoor Biologic Agents: A Review of the Evidence."

26 Noreen Beatley, "Green Housing=Improved Health: A Winning Combination," National Center for Healthy Housing, 2011.

27 Tim K. Takaro, James Krieger, Lin Song, Denise Sharify, and Nancy Beaudet, "The Breathe-Easy Home: The Impact of Asthma-Friendly Home Construction on Clinical Outcomes and Trigger Exposure," *American Journal of Public Health* 101, no. 1 (2011): 55.

28 ANSI/ASHRAE, *Standard 62.2-2013 Ventilation for Acceptable Indoor Air Quality in Low-Rise Residential Buildings*.

29 EPA, "Indoor Air Facts No. 4 (Revised): Sick Building Syndrome," United States Environmental Protection Agency, 1991.

30 Kathleen Kreiss, "The Sick Building Syndrome: Where Is the Epidemiologic Basis?" *American Journal of Public Health* 80, no. 10 (1990): 1172.

31 WHO, "Indoor Air Pollution: Health and Social Impacts of Household Energy."

32 HSE, "Cross Government Group on Gas Safety and Carbon Monoxide (CO) Awareness: Annual Report 2013/14," Health and Safety Executive, 2014; K. Sircar et al., "Carbon Monoxide Poisoning Deaths in the United States, 1999 to 2012," *The American Journal of Emergency Medicine* 33, no. 9 (2015): 1140.

33 ANSI/ASHRAE, *Standard 62.2-2013 Ventilation for Acceptable Indoor Air Quality in Low-Rise Residential Buildings*; WHO, *WHO Guidelines for Indoor Air Quality: Selected Pollutants* (Geneva, Switzerland: WHO Regional Office for Europe, 2010), www.euro.who.int/__data/assets/pdf_file/0009/128169/e94535.pdf.

34 O. Seppänen, "Healthy Buildings From Science to Practice," in *Healthy Buildings 2003– Proceedings of ISIAQ 7th International Conference*, eds. T. K. Wai, C. Sekhar, and D. Cheong (National University of Singapore, 2003): 29-50.

35 ANSI/ASHRAE, *Thermal Environmental Conditions for Human Occupancy*, Standard 55-2013 (Atlanta, GA: ASHRAE), www.ashrae.org/resources--publications/bookstore/standard-55.

36 Ibid.

37 IOM, *Climate Change, the Indoor Environment, and Health*.

38 Sherry Ahrentzen, James Erickson, and Ernesto Fonseca, "Thermal and Health Outcomes of Energy Efficiency Retrofits of Homes of Older Adults," *Indoor Air* 26 (2016): 582-593; Divine T. Novieto and Yi Zhang, "Thermal Comfort Implications of the Aging Effect on Metabolism, Cardiac Output and Body Weight," paper presented at Adapting to Change: New Thinking on Comfort, Windsor, UK, 2010.

39 Yujin Sunwoo, Chinmei Chou, Junko Takeshita, Motoko Murakami, and Yutaka Tochihara, "Physiological and Subjective Responses to Low Relative Humidity in Young and Elderly Men," *Journal of Physiological Anthropology* 25 (2006): 229; Peder Wolkoff and Soren K. Kjaerrgaard, "The Dichotomy of Relative Humidity on Indoor Air Quality," *Environment International* 33, no. 6 (2007): 850.

40 Institute of Medicine, *Climate Change, the Indoor Environment, and Health*.

41 Wargo, *LEED Certification: Where Energy Efficiency Collides With Human Health*, 28.

42 EPA, *Water on Tap: What You Need to Know* (2009); EPA, *EPA Survey Shows $384 Billion Needed for Drinking Water Infrastructure by 2030* (Washington, DC: USEPA), http://yosemite.epa.gov/opa/admpress.nsf/0/F72C2FDC7D61F92085257B800057655F.

43 EPA, *Drinking Water From Household Wells (Publication Id: 5725)* (Washington, DC: USEPA), http://publications.usa.gov/USAPubs.php?PubID=5725.

44 Wargo, *LEED Certification Where Energy Efficiency Collides With Human Health*.

45 David DiLaura, Kevin Houser, Richard Mistrick, and Gary Steffy, *The Lighting Handbook: Reference and Application*, 10th edition (New York: Illuminating Engineering Society of America, 2011).
46 Peter Boyce, Claudia Hunter, and Owen Howlett, *The Benefits of Daylight Through Windows* (Troy, NY: Rensselaer Polytechnic Institute, 2003); Anjali Joseph, *The Impact of Light on Outcomes in Healthcare Settings* (Concord, CA: Center for Healthcare Design, 2006), www.healthdesign.org/sites/default/files/CHD_Issue_Paper2.pdf; Jennifer A. Veitch, *Conclusion: Is Full Spectrum Light the Quality Choice?* (Ottawa, Canada: Institute for Research in Construction, 1993): 112–114.
47 David DiLaura, Kevin Houser, Richard Mistrick, and Gary Steffy, *The Lighting Handbook: Reference and Application*; U.S. Department of Energy, "Lighting for Health: LEDs in the New Age of Illumination," http://apps1.eere.energy.gov/buildings/publications/pdfs/ssl/light_and_health_fs.pdf.
48 Joseph, *The Impact of Light on Outcomes in Healthcare Settings*.
49 Sherry Ahrentzen and Elif Tural, "The Role of Building Design and Interiors in Ageing Actively at Home," *Building Research and Information* 43, no. 5 (2015): 582–601; Kelly Carr et al., "Universal Design: A Step Toward Successful Aging," *Journal of Aging Research* 2013 (2013): 8; Neville Owen et al., "Sedentary Behavior: Emerging Evidence for a New Health Risk," *Mayo Clinic Proceedings* 85, no. 12 (2010): 1138; Jon A. Sanford, *Universal Design as a Rehabilitation Strategy: Design for the Ages* (New York: Springer, 2012).

8

HEALTH AND WELLNESS IN TODAY'S TECHNOLOGICAL SOCIETY

Eugenia Victoria Ellis and Donald L. McEachron

Introduction

Due to advances in medicine, public health and technology,[1] people live longer today than they did 200 years ago[2]—but has the quality of human life kept pace with this longevity? Until the last century, people woke up with the sunrise, went to bed shortly after sunset, and extended the day with candlelight, oil lamps or a fire. By the early twentieth century, electric lighting became common[3] and people could stay awake throughout the night. Today, people experience many light-related disorders and diseases exactly because they can stay awake for 24 hours per day in electrically illuminated indoor environments. Sleep loss is directly related to an increase in inflammatory markers[4] and the effects of sleep deprivation and sleep disorders are associated with various chronic diseases.[5] Yet, lack of sleep is often overlooked or undervalued as a lifestyle risk factor for chronic disease.[6]

Historically, the leading causes of death have changed from the communicable diseases of the nineteenth century to the chronic diseases of the new millennium.[7] Infant mortality was 20 percent a little over a century ago. Another 20 percent of children died before age 5 due to infectious diseases such as smallpox, measles and diphtheria.[8] More children began to survive due to the introduction and widespread use of penicillin and the polio vaccine in the mid-twentieth century.[9] Today, death from chronic diseases is double that of all others combined including infant mortality, nutritional deficiencies and infectious diseases such as HIV/AIDS.[10] It is surprising when we realize that the primary sources of death 100 years ago were contagious diseases, while today it is chronic diseases such as cardiovascular and heart disease, stroke, cancer, type 2 diabetes and respiratory problems.[11] Today, people live longer and many causes of death can be delayed or avoided by lifestyle changes.

The important difference between a chronic disease and a contagious disease is that we can avoid most common chronic diseases by changes in lifestyle and diet.[12]

Many chronic diseases may be caused by a type of inflammation called metaflammation,[13] which is associated with lifestyle and environmental sources[14] that are linked to chronic diseases, including depression and dementia.[15] Anthropogens cause metaflammation and are a result of changes in the built environment due to the industrial revolution and changing lifestyles.[16] Anthropogens incite a low-level immune response to a possible life-threatening situation, which builds up over time into a systemic response by the body. Although a person might have a genetic tendency to a certain chronic disease, early environmental influences can affect the later development of that disease.[17] Chronic disease can be affected by a mismatch between the environment for which one is evolutionarily and genetically programmed and the environment one is born into or is living in.

Evolution and Design

At first glance, cultural/technological changes and biological evolution appear to be vastly different processes and indeed, they are. However, there are similarities as well. Biological evolution and engineering design can result in similar answers to similar questions, for example, the shape of a bird's and an aircraft's wing. The need for timing in computers and other devices, the evolution of biological clocks and concepts underlying information systems are applicable to everything from biological evolution itself, to the rise of social media, to how genetic systems function to database design and finally, to information processing in the human brain. Additionally, engineering design and biological evolution must deal with both ultimate functions and proximate mechanisms, an ultimate function being the overall purpose of a device and the proximate mechanisms the means by which that overall purpose is achieved.

However, there are significant differences as well. The ultimate goal of biological evolution is to preserve and propagate genes—organisms could be considered as a mere means to the end of spreading genes. When engineering the built environment, the ultimate goal is the health, well-being and productivity of the people who will live there. While engineering design calculates measurable results, biological evolution is based upon errors that randomly occur in the genetic material. These errors may or may not turn out to have an advantage. Not every possible must design or advantage arises in evolution that could be rationally expected. Biological evolution is also relatively slow compared with the pace of cultural/technological change. Thus, aspects of physiology, and even behavior, that might have been useful in our ancestors' environments may or may not have changed to suit today's world.

How does this impact design? What it means, in essence, is that we must design for humans that are only partially adapted to the current environment. Also, this mismatch between biology and culture is likely to get worse as the rate of technological change increases. Thus, there must be a kind of evolutionary element, an almost irrational design perspective, to the creation of artificial structures in order to fit those structures to the irrational/evolutionary elements of human nature.

An important aspect of our ancestors' environment—all the way back to the origins of cellular life—is the gradual alternation of light and darkness generated by the Earth's rotation. For both engineering design and evolutionary reasons, this environmental condition has shaped the evolution of all living systems and has profound implications for artificial environments.

Biological Rhythms: Timing Is Everything

Biological rhythms, put simply, are regular periodic variations in any biological system. Everyone is familiar with some biological rhythms, such as the cardiac cycle, breathing and walking, but few recognize that rhythms are a fundamental characteristic of all living processes. Rhythms are found everywhere, from cycles in biochemical reactions to subcellular rhythms in mitochondria to cell division cycles, as well as the neural oscillations measured by electroencephalograms (EEG), the pulsing release of hormones, 24-hour sleep-wake rhythms, menstrual cycles, annual rhythms in births and so on. The human body is comprised of hundreds of rhythms with a variety of frequencies.

Why so many rhythms with so many frequencies? Is there a deeper underlying purpose or are human rhythms merely a legacy effect of some prior evolutionary circumstance? This latter hypothesis seems unlikely in the face of the observation that all living systems—not just humans—incorporate rhythms into their fundamental operations. As science continues to investigate the role of rhythms in living systems, a number of fundamental reasons for their evolution have emerged. These include:

1. *The need for timing mechanisms in complex, goal-oriented devices.* When a car is tuned, one important aspect to regulate is the timing so the engine parts function at the proper time with respect to each other. Living systems are exceedingly complex, goal-oriented systems and require timing systems that are based upon oscillations or rhythms so that all parts work well with each other.
2. *Feedback control systems are inherently oscillatory.* Biological systems incorporate various feedback control systems and these systems have a fundamental tendency to oscillate.
3. *Output systems are often rhythmic in nature.* Pumping blood, breathing, walking—all of these are examples of output behavior or physiology that is inherently cyclic. It should not be surprising that the control systems for such rhythmic outputs—the heart or central pattern generators in the brainstem and spinal cord—are also oscillatory.
4. *Finally, the Earth's rotation and revolution around the sun create major and predictable environmental fluctuations to which Earth's organisms must adapt.*

The first two reasons listed above are common to both engineering design and biological evolution. The fact that organisms use oscillations to time critical events may be partially due to evolutionary forces taking advantage of the rhythmic nature of feedback systems, but the need for timing is fundamental in both engineering design and biological evolution. The third reason is also part evolution and part fundamental, as can be seen by the rhythmic nature of the internal combustion engine leading to wheel rotations in ground vehicles. The last reason—day/night and seasonal cycles—is not fundamental to design per se and therein lies a problem. Our devices may not have been designed with daily and/or seasonal rhythms, but our bodies have evolved oscillations to adapt to those rhythms and this disconnect leads to artificial environments and societal demands that do not facilitate, and may actually interfere with, our daily and seasonal patterns.

Why do we care? If daily—referred to as circadian rhythms—are not fundamental to complex designs, could we as humans dispense with them? After all, we are not living outside, subject to the vast environmental changes associated with day and night—if we want light at night, we can simply generate it. We are not dependent on the sun, so why should we be concerned?

Remember that the human body is composed of hundreds of biological rhythms with a variety of frequencies. One of the fundamental functions of these rhythms is to coordinate multiple activities and cycles so the body can function optimally. And this is not merely a biological requirement but rather a constraint on any complex, goal-oriented system. Thus, this requirement cannot simply be dismissed. The problem we face is that circadian rhythmicity has evolved, in part, to coordinate an organism's various rhythms to maintain internal temporal order.

To fully appreciate the situation, consider a symphony orchestra. When arriving before a performance the musicians are tuning up and the result could not really be described as music—a cacophony of noise is a more appropriate description. What converts this noise to music? The conductor provides temporal order to the various components of the orchestra. The human body is a far more complex system of rhythms but nevertheless has a conductor—a master pacemaker or biological clock that provides temporal order to the system. This pacemaker runs at a frequency of about 1 cycle every 24.2 hours and is known as the circadian clock (located in an area of the brain called the suprachiasmatic nuclei of the hypothalamus or SCN).

The SCN accomplish two major tasks. The SCN help confer an internal temporal order onto the various rhythms of the human body and mind. Also, the SCN positions these rhythms within the Earth's cycle of day and night so that physiological and behavioral processes occur at the appropriate times—activity during the day and sleep at night. Since the actual inherent rhythm of the SCN does not exactly match that of the day/night cycle (24.2 vs. 24), the SCN need to be reset every day to maintain the correct positioning, which is done by the rising and setting sun through our exposure to the right intensities and wavelengths of light at the right times of day. Everyone's behavioral and physiological activities are regulated by rhythms of varying frequencies that are tied to a consistent daily pattern run by a biological clock synchronized to the sun's day/night cycle.

What characterizes this day/night cycle? A light intensity that increases gradually (sunrise), then displays a powerful, sustained intensity (daylight) followed by a gradual decrease (sunset) and then a prolonged period of profound darkness (night). In addition to light intensity, the color of light changes from red-yellow at sunrise/sunset to blue-white at mid-day and near blackness at night. In terms of illuminance levels, light intensity might vary from 34,000 lux at mid-day to barely 1 lux at sunrise/sunset to 0.0001 lux under a starry night (see Figure 8.1).

While details vary depending on location and habitat, biological systems have evolved in environments which provide gradual illuminance changes covering 6–9 orders of magnitude.

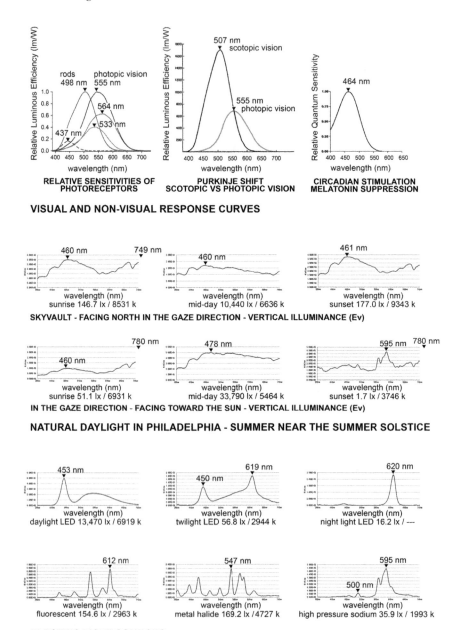

FIGURE 8.1 Spectral Response Curves for Vision, Non-visual Information and Light

How do most circadian clocks synchronize with the day/night cycle? The primary mechanism involves a pattern of specific phase shifts. Circadian systems vary in light-sensitivity across their cycles. To synchronize (a process called entrainment) to day/night cycles, circadian systems typically undergo a repeating pattern of phase shifts which align the internal circadian clock with the external environmental cycle. Light exposure at times other than those that promote synchronization can shift rhythms dramatically and increase the chances of both external (mismatch between the external environment and internal rhythms) and internal desynchronization.[18]

To make matters even more complex, for many circadian systems, including the human circadian clock, the internal frequencies of the clock are based upon the light intensity to which the organism is exposed. This involves both absolute intensity and duration. Thus, the frequency expressed by the human circadian clock differs with respect to seasonal changes in photoperiod and alters our daily rhythms. For example, during the summer, the period of the underlying circadian rhythm becomes longer and is expressed in a phase delay of the entrained rhythms; in winter, the opposite occurs and results in phase advances. These changes can trigger significant behavioral and physiological alterations, exemplified in the human condition known as Seasonal Affective Disorder (SAD).

Anatomy of the Visual and Non-Visual Eye

When light enters the eye, the body responds in three ways: object recognition or vision, the internal and external synchronization of biological rhythms and a direct stimulating effect on alertness and performance.[19] It is important to understand how we see and how the eye responds to light to understand how the body responds to light (Figure 8.2). If we can understand how the body responds to light, then we can know how to go about designing the indoor lighting environment.

People see when light enters the eye through a responsive, open pupil and passes through the lens. The lens and pupil work together to focus the light on the back of the retina at the fovea where cone cells are densely packed to provide fine visual acuity and color discrimination.

There are three kinds of cone cells responsible for color vision: red or long-wavelength (L—564 nm peak), green or medium-wavelength (M—533 nm peak) and blue or short-wavelength (S—437 nm peak) (see Figure 8.1). Color is understood by the brain as a comparison function between the L, M and S cone cells. The cones are less dense away from the fovea where they are intermingled with the rods. The rods (498 nm peak) are primarily responsible for peripheral vision and provide information about contrast and movement, which is why we respond quicker when an object comes into our peripheral vision than when we stare directly at it.

The cones are most active in medium and high light levels and function at higher *photopic* levels of illumination. The rods become overwhelmed with high light levels, but respond well at low light levels and function best at lower *scotopic* levels. As the general environmental brightness drops, the cones become less effective and it becomes difficult to discern fine details and colors. When we move

RETINAL GANGLION CELLS

2.4–3 million cells
convey visual signals to the optic nerve
contribute to vision
stimulate pupillary light reflex

CONES

6 million cells
function well in daylight
contain three types of photosensitive pigments for color: S, M, L
responsible for color discrimination
densely packed in the fovea
high visual acuity and spatial resolution

ipRGCs

1–3% of retinal ganglion cells
contain the photopigment melanopsin
sensitive to blue light
non-image forming functions
melatonin production

RODS

120 million cells
function in low light
contain one type of photosensitive pigment in the blue spectrum
confer achromatic vision
intermingled with cones in the retina
good for peripheral vision, contrast and movement

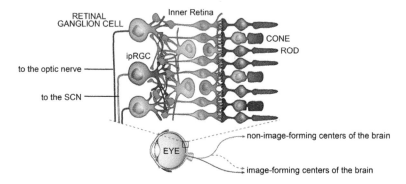

FIGURE 8.2 Anatomy of the Eye: Light in Layers

Source: Adapted by permission from Macmillan Publishers Ltd: [NATURE] (Corie Lok, "Seeing Without Seeing," 469/7330, pp. 284–285), copyright (2011)

from natural daylight to the indoor environment or from daylight to darkness, our eyes adapt to changing illumination levels. This transition requires that our eyes shift from photopic vision toward scotopic vision so that both rods and cones are contributing to vision. This intermediate lighting level is characteristic of most indoor environments and is the *mesopic* level when both cones and rods contribute to vision.

This change in spectral sensitivity is known as the Purkinje shift (see Figure 8.1). When the light intensity begins to drop toward darkness, vision begins to shift from cone vision to rod vision. The peak of the photopic response curve is at around 555 nm and the scotopic peak is at 507 nm. Even though illumination levels are lower at the peak of scotopic vision, since rods are so light-sensitive, the relative lighting level appears to be over twice as bright. During scotopic vision, any light will blind the rods and will appear very bright, such as light filtering through a window at night. It is very possible this light may alter rhythms and/or stimulate arousal to cause temporal disorder.

A third type of photoreceptor is the retinal ganglion cell, which is located in the inner retina and sends signals from the rods and cones to the brain (see Figure 8.2).

Light to these cells causes the pupil to open or close and non-visual photoneu-ral responses (circadian, neuroendocrine and neurobehavioral regulation). A small subset (~ 1–3 percent) of these cells is called the intrinsically photosensitive Ret-inal Ganglion Cells (ipRGCs), which has an absorption peak at approximately 480 nm.[20] As it turns out, there are several pathways for light to take on its way to the brain. Visual information can be taken by the optic nerve to be processed by the image-forming centers of the brain. Or, non-visual information can be transmitted by other pathways to the suprachiasmatic nuclei (SCN), which relay signals throughout the nervous system to provide information regarding time of day and ambient levels of light and darkness. The pineal gland receives these non-visual signals from the SCN, which regulate its production and secretion of the hormone melatonin. Melatonin, among other things, helps the body to sleep. Mela-tonin production is greatest at night and lowest during the day for optimal circadian function. Its production is suppressed by blue-white light[21] with a peak at around 464nm,[22] which closely matches the 480 nm ipRGC peak (see Figure 8.1).

Rod light response peaks sharply at 498 nm in the blue spectrum and responds very little to red light (see Figure 8.1). This leads to some interesting phenomena. If mesopic vision is desirable, for example, high-acuity vision at night without circa-dian rhythm disruption, then red-adapted vision is a solution. This can be achieved by using red light or by wearing red goggles.[23] This way the cones receive enough light for high-acuity photopic vision, for example reading, without disrupting our circadian rhythms. Similarly, red goggles can block the blue light of various elec-tronic media. Rods are not affected by the red light because they are not sensitive to long-wavelength light. On the other hand, vision will have very little color contrast so what we see will appear in shades of gray, blue will become black and objects that are yellow will seem to disappear. Even dim light at night without a red filter is not desirable. Since rod vision is shifted toward the blue spectrum, even a tiny bit of light can transmit non-visual information to reduce melatonin production.

Do Rhythms Really Matter?

Biological rhythms are key elements controlling physiological activities. Operating at various frequencies, these rhythms must be coordinated to achieve optimum health and well-being. Due to the impact and predictability of the day/night cycle, evolution has equipped all eukaryotic organisms—including humans—with pow-erful circadian clocks that serve to both regulate these internal rhythms and align them with the geophysical cycle of day and night. Although multi-faceted, the most effective means of attaining this alignment (entraining) is through the appropriate applications of light and darkness through the eyes.

Two major implications of these observations are: 1) inappropriate application of light or darkness will disrupt internal rhythms and temporal order; and 2) such disruptions will be detrimental to human health, well-being and productivity. Are these implications actually true?

They are indeed true. Although it is impossible to cover all the data currently available, accidental human experiments involving shift work and travel across time zones, confirmed through specific animal experimentation have conclusively demonstrated that disrupting circadian rhythms and internal temporal order negatively impacts both behavior and physiology.[24] Some of these adverse effects include an increased risk for cancer,[25] changes in brain function,[26] insulin resistance and obesity[27] and greater incidents of cardiovascular disease[28]—all chronic diseases. These effects are heightened with special needs populations whose physiological systems are already under more pronounced stresses such as children with autism spectrum disorder, older adults with dementia and homeless individuals. In short, poor temporal hygiene generated by disrupting circadian rhythms leads to poor health outcomes and a decrease in the quality of human life. And what is one of the primary means of disrupting human circadian rhythms? Irregular schedules enabled by inappropriate electric lighting.

Chronobioengineering the Indoor Environment

Chronobioengineering uses knowledge gleaned from the natural world out of which we evolved to guide design of the built world into which we find ourselves living today. While design regulations for indoor lighting focus on light levels for specific visual tasks, designers still need to consider the possible adverse health effects of electric lighting that could disrupt the building occupant's temporal hygiene. Although lighting design alone cannot solve the problems generated by our modern 24/7 technological society, it might reduce its negative results.

Question—can lighting in our indoor environments be designed to promote temporal health without abandoning the flexibility 24-hour light provides? The answer is maybe, but there will have to be some changes. The retina and SCN cannot distinguish between electric and natural daylight if the light is of similar wavelength and intensity. This represents both a disadvantage and advantage; a disadvantage if we design the indoor lighting environment without considering wavelength and intensity, but an advantage if we know how light impacts the circadian system.

In terms of timing, both mathematical models of biological rhythms and experimental observations of circadian rhythms in organisms indicate that a gradual onset and offset of light intensity will generate a far more powerful and sustained synchronization than light pulses or even a typical square-wave approach. A typical square-wave lighting system (such as turning lights on at 6 am and off again at 6 pm generating a LD (Light/Dark) 12/12 cycle) is not optimal for entrainment of circadian rhythms. The signals generated by this LD cycle are perceived by the circadian clock not as a single timing signal but rather as a mixture of many sine and cosine waveforms. These conflicting signals reduce the efficacy of the LD cycle as a synchronizing agent.[29]

A more appropriate sinusoidal light intensity waveform with suitable wavelengths means a gradual onset/offset lighting environment that changes wavelength and intensity similarly to the rising and setting sun with sustained light intensity throughout the day. This is like the lighting environment from which humans evolved. Light intensity varies dramatically throughout the day, drastically changing in intensity when measured in the gaze direction or vertical illuminance (E_v) (see Figure 8.1). Natural daylight from the sky vault is characteristic for most of the outdoors, which does greatly differ in intensity than if we gaze horizontally toward the sun (not at the sun). The graphs indicate a peak in long wavelengths during sunrise and sunset when the rays of the sun cut horizontally through the Earth's atmosphere. How light is measured is important. In lighting design, light is characteristically measured by horizontal illuminance (E_h), or the measure of light on a horizontal surface, which is facing upwards. People rarely stare up at the ceiling. Lighting should be designed for where people will be looking, whether across while seated at a desk or dining table, down at the floor while walking, or up at the ceiling while in bed or a dentist's chair.

In terms of perception, designers can take advantage of the different absorption spectra of photoreception involving circadian rhythms and vision. If current studies by the dLUX light lab at Drexel University are confirmed, dim red light will allow for activities during the dark phase of lighting while having little or no impact on the circadian system.[30] Therefore, absolute darkness may not be needed to avoid circadian disruption, which supports the notion of circadian design in lighting systems for temporal health.

Human vision is normally better with daylight than electric lighting. This is largely due to the higher intensity of natural daylight and its better color rendering index, two properties of light that electric lighting seeks to copy.[31] Even though we tend to prefer the light levels of natural daylight, especially as provided by the mid-day sun, we do not always adjust our indoor lighting environment to follow the natural changes in daylight in its daily change from the rising sun to the mid-day sun to the setting sun.[32] Unfortunately, in order to reduce heat from the sun in warm climates, we often shade our windows to keep out the light and use electric light instead to see, when we could be controlling the natural daylight to both see and boost our circadian systems.

Guidelines for Environmental Illumination

Natural daylight is the part of the electromagnetic spectrum seen by the human eye and processed as visual and non-visual information. Research has shown that people working in natural sunlight are more productive, more effective and happier than those who work under traditional electric light[33] and that indoor lighting has increasingly become a public health issue.[34] In June 2012 at the American Medical Association (AMA) annual meeting, their House of Delegates declared that light at night results in adverse health outcomes. Furthermore, the Council on Science and Public Health recognized that exposure to excessive light at night, including extended use of various electronic media, can disrupt sleep or exacerbate sleep disorders. They recommended that the AMA support research into new lighting technologies and the use of lighting at home and at work to minimize circadian disruption and provide light for daily activities.[35]

It is easy to maximize natural daylight in the design of the indoor environment for health and wellness. For building design, 1) use large areas of north-facing glass and 2) provide many windows on the other three façades with sun control devices to shade the glass from radiant heat while redirecting natural daylight deep into the building interior. For interior design, use natural illumination together with electric lighting to provide ambient light while controlling glare with window treatments. The use of natural daylight to guide the design of a building is a rather old, yet effective, technology that predates the Roman atrium. In the lighting industry, electric lighting has changed greatly over the past 10 years from the use of either electric-filament or gas lamps in light fixtures to the light-emitting diode (LED) lamp, or the integrated LED luminaire with no lamp at all but LEDs integrated within the fixture.[36]

Compared with either electric-filament or gas lamps, LEDs can most closely match the full spectrum of natural daylight in color and intensity, can be tuned to mimic the rising, setting and noontime sun, and can provide red light at night (see Figure 8.1). In addition, the LED waveform has continuous variability like natural daylight, while the waveform of the gas-lamp is jagged and discontinuous. Colors of the various peaks of a gas lamp light source can sum to equal white, but there are gaps in the spectrum, which is likely why human vision is more comfortable with daylight than gas-lamp lighting. The continuity of the LED waveform holds the promise of more closely matching the comfort of natural daylight. Research is underway at the dLUX light lab to measure the eye's response to the different waveforms of electric light with respect to comfort and to confirm the wavelength ranges for melatonin production and/or suppression.

Depending on jurisdiction, various codes govern the required light levels for indoor lighting at the local, state and national levels. Also, the Illuminating Engineering Society provides recommended practices for various user groups. What these guidelines do not take into consideration is the changing physiology of the aging human body or special needs populations. For example, aging decreases pupil area and reduces lens light transmission which blocks blue light and results in progressive loss of circadian photoreception. The amount of light reaching the human retina decreases about 1 percent per year. This means that if a 10-year-old child's retina receives 100 percent of available light from the environment, then the 90-year-old adult retina receives only 10 percent of that available light. This drastically limits the older adult's circadian system from receiving the light it needs for photoentrainment[37] and is likely why studies recommend blue-shifted light of 6500k with lighting levels as high as 2500 lux for older adults,[38] for at least a portion of the day.

Conclusion

Lighting the indoor environment considers the use of the space together with the particular needs of the person who will be occupying the space and his/her special needs. For optimal health and well-being in interior architecture, environmental illumination supports improved circadian photoreception by using natural daylight together with electric lighting that mimics light from the sun and the solar day.

Acknowledgements

The authors thank the American Society of Interior Designers Foundation for their gracious support of Drexel University's dLUX light lab research on light and health.

Notes

1 Jim Oeppen and James W. Vaupel, "Broken Limits to Life Expectancy," *Science* 296 (May 10, 2002): 1029–1030.

2 James C. Riley, *Rising Life Expectancy: A Global History* (Cambridge: Cambridge University Press, 2001), 243.

3 Ernest Freebert, *The Age of Edison: Electric Light and the Invention of Modern America* (New York: The Penguin Group, 2014).

4 Jane E. Ferrie, Mika Kivim"aki, Tasnime N. Akbaraly et al., "Associations Between Change in Sleep Duration and Inflammation: Findings on C-Reactive Protein and Interleukin 6 in the Whitehall II Study," *The American Journal of Epidemiology* 178, no. 6 (2013): 956–961; Sarosh J. Motivala, "Sleep and Inflammation: Psychoneuroimmunology in the Context of Cardiovascular Disease," *Annals of Behavioral Medicine* 42, no. 2 (2011): 141–152.

5 Harvey R. Colten and Bruce M. Altevogt, eds. *Sleep Disorders and Sleep Deprivation: An Unmet Public Health Problem* (Washington, DC: National Academies Press, 2006).

6 Mary E. Wells and Bradley V. Vaughn, "Poor Sleep Challenging the Health of a Nation," *The Neurodiagnostic Journal* 52, no. 3 (2012): 233–249.

7 John W. Sanders, Greg S. Fuhrer, Mark D. Johnson, and Mark S. Riddle, "The Epidemiological Transition: The Current Status of Infectious Diseases in the Developed World Versus the Developing World," *Science Progress* 91, no. 1 (2008): 1–38.

8 Alexandra Minna Stern and Howard Markel, "The History of Vaccines and Immunization: Familiar Patterns, New Challenges," *Health Affairs* 24, no. 3 (May/Jun 2005): 611–21.

9 Alan Hinman, "Landmark Perspective: Mass Vaccination Against Polio," *JAMA* 251, no. 22 (1984): 2994–2996.

10 World Health Organization, "Part Two. The Urgent Need for Action, Chapter One. Chronic Diseases: Causes and Health Impact," *Chronic diseases and health promotion*, www.who.int/chp/chronic_disease_report/part2_ch1/en/index1.html.

11 World Health Organization, www.who.int/chp/chronic_disease_report/part2_ch1/en/index4.html.

12 Goodarz Danaei Eric L. Ding, Dariush Mozaffarian, Ben Taylor, Jürgen Rehm,, Christopher J. L. Murray, Majid Ezzati, "The Preventable Causes of Death in the United States: Comparative Risk Assessment of Dietary, Lifestyle, and Metabolic Risk Factors," *PLoS Medicine* 8(1): doi: 10.1371/annotation/0ef47acd-9dcc-4296-a897-872d182cde57 (April 2009).

13 Gokhan S. Hotamisligil, "Inflammation and Metabolic Disorders," *Nature* 444, no. 7121 (2006): 860–867.

14 Rusian Medzhitov, "Origin and Physiological Roles of Inflammation," *Nature* 454, no. 7203 (2008): 428–435.

15 Peter Libby, "Inflammatory Mechanisms: The Molecular Basis of Inflammation and Disease," *Nutrition Reviews* 65, no. 12 (2007): S140–S146.

16 Garry Egger, "In Search of a "Germ Theory" Equivalent for Chronic Disease," *Preventing Chronic Disease* 9, no. 11 (2012): 1–7.

17 Garry Egger and John Dixon, "Beyond Obesity and Lifestyle: A Review of 21st Century Chronic Disease Determinants," *BioMed Research International* (2014), Article ID 731685, 12 pages, http://dx.doi.org/10.1155/2014/731685.

18 Donald L. McEachron, "Disruption of Internal Temporal Order," in *Chronobioengineering: Introduction to Biological Rhythms With Applications*, Vol. 1 (San Francisco, CA: Morgan Claypool, 2012): 141-151.

19 Fabien Perrin, Philippe Peigneux, Sonia Fuchs, Stephen Verhaeghe, Steven Laureys, Benita Middleton, Christian Degueldre, Guy del Fiore, Gilles Vanderwalle, Evelyne Balteau, Robert Poirier, Vincent Moreau, Andre Luxen, Pierre Maquet, and Derk-Jan Dijk, "Nonvisual Responses to Light Exposure in the Human Brain," *Current Biology* 14 (2004): 1842–1846.

20 David M. Berson, "Phototransduction in Ganglion-Cell Photoreceptors," *Pflügers Archiv-European Journal of Physiology* 454, no. 5 (2007): 849–855.

21 Alfred J. Lewy, Thomas A. Wehr, Frederick K. Goodwin, David A. Newsome, and S. P. Markey, "Light Suppresses Melatonin Secretion in Humans," *Science* 210, no. 4475 (December 12, 1980): 1267–1269.

22 George C. Brainard, John P. Hanifin, Jeffrey M. Greeson, Brenda Byrne, Gena Glickman, Edward Gerner, and Mark D. Rollag, "Action Spectrum for Melatonin Regulation in Humans: Evidence for a Novel Circadian Photoreceptor," *Journal of Neuroscience* 21, no. 16 (August 15, 2001): 6405–6412.

23 Masahiko Ayaki, Atsuhiko Hattori, Yusuke Maruyama, Masaki Nakano, Michitaka Yoshimura, Momoko Kitazawa, Kazuno Negishi, and Kazuo Tsubota, "Protective Effect of Blue-light Shield Eyewear for Adults Against Light Pollution from Self-luminous Devices Used at Night," *Chronobiology International* 33, no. 1 (2016): 134–139.

24 McEachron, *Chronobioengineering*.

25 Steven S. Coughlin and Selina A. Smith, "The Impact of the Natural, Social, Built and Policy Environments on Breast Cancer," *Journal of Environment and Health Science* 1, no. 3 (2015), doi:10.15436/2378-6841.15.020; Daniel Guitierrez and Joshua Arbesman, "Circadian Dysrhythmias, Physiological Aberrations and the Link to Skin Cancer," *International Journal of Molecular Sciences* 17, no. 621 (2016), doi:10.3390/ijms17050621.

26 Ilia N. Karatsoreos et al., "Disruption of Circadian Clocks Has Ramifications for Metabolism, Brain and Behavior," *PNAS* 108, no. 4 (2010): 1657–1662.

27 Shu-qun Shi et al., "Circadian Disruption Leads to Insulin Resistance and Obesity," *Current Biology* 23 (2013): 372–381.

28 Sirimon Reutrakul and Kristen L. Knutson, "Consequences of Circadian Disruption on Cardiometabolic Health," *Sleep Medicine Clinic* 10 (2015): 455–468.

29 McEachron, *Chronobioengineering*, Chapter 6.

30 Eugenia V. Ellis, Donald L. McEachron, Elizabeth W. Gonzalez, and David A. Kratzer, "Red Light at Night to Enhance Cognitive Functioning for Society's Special Needs Groups," *Societal Challenges: Proceedings of the 2016 ARCC/EAAE International Conference on Architectural Research* (Lisbon: Taylor & Francis, 2016).

31 Myriam B. C. Aries, Mariëlle P. J. Aarts, Joost van Hoof, "Daylight and Health: A Review of the Evidence and Consequences for the Built Environment," *Lighting Research Technology* 47 (2015): 6–27.

32 Guy R. Newsham, Myriam B. C. Aries, Simona Mancini, and G. Faye, "Individual Control of Electric Lighting in a Daylit Space," *Lighting Research and Technology* 40 (2008): 25–41.

33 Fabien Perrin et al., "Nonvisual Responses to Light Exposure in the Human Brain," *Current Biology* 14 (2004): 1842–1846.

34 Stephen M. Pauley, "Lighting for the Human Circadian Clock: Recent Research Indicates That Lighting Has Become a Public Health Issue," *Medical Hypotheses* 63 (2004): 588–596.

35 David Blask, George Brainard, Ronald Gibbons, Steven Lockley, Richard Stevens, and Mario Motta, "Light Pollution: Adverse Health Effects of Nighttime Lighting," *Action of the AMA House of Delegates 2012 Annual Meeting: Council on Science and Public Health Report* 4 (A-12), 25 pages.

36 Eugenia V. Ellis, Donald L. McEachron, Elizabeth W. Gonzalez, and David A. Kratzer, "EBD Using Daylight-Mimicking LEDs for Improved Health Outcomes in Older Adults at St Francis," in *Proceedings of the 2014 ARCC/EAAE International Conference on Architectural Research,* David Rockwood and Marja Sarvimäki, eds. (Mānoa: University of Hawai'i, 2014): 275–285.

37 Patricia L. Turner and Martin A. Mainster, "Circadian Photoreception: Ageing and the Eye's Important Role in Systemic Health," *British Journal of Ophthalmology* 92 (2008): 1439–1444.

38 Joost Van Hoof, Mariëlle P. J. Aarts, C. G. Rense, and Antonius M. C. Schoutens, "Ambient Bright Light in Dementia: Effects on Behavior and Circadian Rhythmicity," *Building and Environment* 44 (2009): 146–155; Marianne M. Sinoo, Joost van Hoof, and Helianthe S. M. Kort, "Light Conditions for Older Adults in the Nursing Home: Assessment of Environmental Illuminances and Colour Temperature," *Building and Environment* 46 (2011): 1917–1927.

9

SALUTOGENIC DESIGN FOR BIRTH

Maralyn J. Foureur and J. Davis Harte

Introduction

This chapter focuses on one relatively small aspect of design thinking and practice that concerns the building of just one room, the space and place for birth. The argument we present is that much of current design thinking in this area falls far short of what is needed to support the ongoing health and well-being of the population this space is meant to serve: relatively young, healthy, pregnant women engaged in the salutogenic, physiologically normal activity of giving birth.

This designed space impacts on the way birth happens which has lifelong consequences for women, their babies and their families.[1] We also know that the design of the birth space has a powerful influence on the people who work there and influences their care-giving practices and interactions with women and their supporters.

We suggest that the design and construction of current birth environments is predicated on a belief that birth is a dangerous and risk-filled undertaking; the woman's body is unreliable in its role of protecting the unborn child and safely delivering it into waiting hands. The resulting principles underpinning birth-space design are therefore oriented towards heightened surveillance of the woman and her baby and ease of access to the woman's body to ensure immediate diagnosis of problems and transfer to an operating room to safely complete the birth process. The design consequences are architectural structures and artifacts that communicate suspicion and fear.

More than a decade of research into the relationship between architecture and neuroscience has provided a wealth of information that can now be applied to establish salutogenic design principles that focus on the positive impact of design on human health. In this chapter we offer insights into how the body/mind of the woman giving birth is impacted upon by the birth environment. We suggest how a salutogenic design approach may result in radical new spaces that provide positive experiences for women, their babies and supporters and their care providers.

Outline of the Chapter Content

The chapter begins by exploring the concepts of 'salutogenesis' and 'pathogenesis' in order to reveal the way society's view of childbirth has resulted in a particular set of familiar features in the architecture and design of birth units. A predominant pathological design inspiration is revealed in the description of common features that emerged following the historical 1930s move of birth from home to hospital—design features still in evidence today. Research describing correlations between place of birth and birth outcomes presents a plausible consequence of these pathogenically inspired design decisions. An understanding of the plausibility of such consequences is offered through exploring current knowledge of the neurophysiology of labor and birth and women's responses to stressful experiences. Subsequently, research investigating the impact of the birth environment on a woman's chosen birth companions and her care providers is presented in order to support the knowledge prevalent in other fields, that all bodies respond to cues in the environment which impact on their sense of well-being. The chapter concludes by offering a way forward for the salutogenic design of birth spaces that enable the laboring woman's neurophysiology to remain optimal and undisturbed.

Word restrictions have led us to include a select range of references. Please see the following sites where you will find further additional references and resources (www.uts.edu.au/research-and-teaching/our-research/midwifery-child-family-health/research/projects/birth-unit-design; www.worldhealthdesign.com).

Salutogenesis and Pathogenesis

Salutogenesis is a term describing an approach to health that focuses on factors that actively promote health and well-being, instead of the predominant approach to health, which focuses on pathogenesis—factors that cause disease, or are responses to illness/injury.[2] Salutogenesis proposes that optimal health for each individual is sustained through a dynamic ability to adapt to life's changing circumstances. This ability arises from the combination of three resources that make up a 'Sense of Coherence': 'manageability' which is the capacity to maintain homeostasis and physical function; 'comprehensibility' which is the capacity to understand and negotiate the contexts in which we find ourselves; and resources that enrich a sense of 'meaningfulness', constituted as the desires, causes and concerns that give us the need to resist illness and disease in the first place.[3] An inability to adapt to life's experiences can result from the ubiquitous challenges to these resources that exert a continuous disintegrative force allowing physical or mental illness to overcome a person.

A salutogenic approach to childbirth conceptualizes women's sense of coherence resources as: the capacity to grow a healthy baby and to give birth in a straightforward way utilizing the neurophysiological abilities inherent in the healthy, life-giving act of human reproduction (manageability); having an understanding of the narrative that women possess an innate and powerful ability to give birth, and can therefore anticipate experiencing a sense of trust, control and safety during the process (comprehensibility); and the affirming and enriching sense of purpose in producing a new member of the family, society and culture, to fulfill future dreams (meaningfulness).

Resources that enhance one's sense of coherence can be liberated through a salutogenic approach to architecture and design, thereby enabling a resistance to illness,[4] or in the case of the birthing woman, enabling a resistance to the need for pharmaceutical or operative procedures to safely complete the birth process.

However, the architecture and design of the majority of modern maternity settings are replete with examples of the ubiquitous challenges to one's sense of coherence. This chapter argues these challenges have arisen because of a pathogenic view of childbirth that evolved in the early twentieth century when childbirth moved from home to hospital in what has been referred to as the largest uncontrolled and unevaluated experiment in the Western world.[5]

Evolution of Current Birth Unit Design

In most industrialized countries, women did not begin to move into institutional birth spaces until the 1930s. Until then, home was considered the safest place for birth and where women's family and friends provided support and midwives and doctors were invited to attend. Hospitals were places traditionally reserved for the sick and dying. The institutional spaces women encountered in hospital were initially shared spaces with birthing women in neighboring beds. Women birthed without family support, in the care and control of professional strangers. With increasing use of interventions such as forceps for delivering the baby and chloroform for anesthetizing the mother, birth was moved into operating-room-style single rooms, where it remained for decades. Calls for 'humanizing birth' were made in the 1960s seeking more home-like birth rooms and the inclusion of the woman's husband or supportive companions.[6] Some modifications were made with material decoration of the space and an invitation for supporters to attend, but fundamental design change to the birth room did not occur. The high narrow bed, similar to an operating room table, remained in the central position in the room and the large overhead light remained positioned above it. Other apparatus that might be needed to monitor the progress of the woman's labor or the well-being of her baby remained in the room, all of it in plain view.

The continued call for 'humanizing birth' saw the later evolution of birth centers, either attached to hospital labor wards, or as freestanding buildings. Birth centers were based on fulfilling the need for a more domestic aesthetic in the birth space as well as access to some of the pain relief options available in hospitals. Birth centers continue in many locations but access is usually strictly limited to an ever-decreasing number of women who are considered to be at 'low risk' of obstetric complications.

Impact of Currently Designed Spaces on the Woman: Place of Birth Matters

It is clear that place of birth matters. In a UK survey conducted by the National Childbirth Trust, nine out of ten women felt that the physical environment influenced how easy or difficult it was to give birth.[7] These views are supported by well-conducted studies of women's experiences and birth outcomes in differently designed locations for birth. A prospective cohort study of birth outcomes for 64,538 low-risk women conducted in England revealed there were fewer obstetric interventions with no impact on baby outcomes when women birthed in 'out-of-hospital settings' such as midwife-led birth centers (freestanding or attached to a hospital), compared with obstetric hospital settings.[8] Studies have also been conducted in Canada,[9] the Netherlands[10] and elsewhere with similar findings. Place of birth is associated with different outcomes with less intervention in out-of-hospital settings.

Many factors vary depending on the place of birth and any of these may have played a part in the findings of these studies. Characteristics include the architecture and aesthetics of the birth space as well as models of care and procedures available in the space. In out-of-hospital settings one or two midwives provide one-to-one care for each woman throughout her pregnancy and birth experience.[11] In most hospital settings, this model of care is rarely available with women receiving care from many different health professionals. A recent systematic review of 15 randomized controlled trials (RCTs) of the one-to-one model revealed that women received fewer interventions with no negative impact on baby outcomes.[12] However, in observational studies of one-to-one midwives' practices in many settings it is apparent that no matter the location for birth, these midwives alter the environment in an attempt to make it appear less medical, more home-like and therefore potentially less stressful for the woman.[13] Therefore, it may not be the model of care alone contributing to improved outcomes seen in RCTs. The architecture and aesthetics of the birth space are also critical elements to consider.

Surveillance Rooms

The following illustrations comparing hospital and out-of-hospital settings reveal the design features and artifacts that may positively or negatively influence the user's experience. The hospital birth rooms in Figures 9.1a and 9.1b are typical, current examples of the enduring design established in the first half of the twentieth century, described elsewhere as bed-centric, surveillance rooms.[14] The equipment located next to the bed indicates the need for continuous surveillance of the baby's heartbeat with a cardio-toco-graphic (CTG) machine in a prominent position. The infant resuscitaire located beside the CTG machine is a constant reminder that in this setting, birth is regarded as a situation of high risk for the baby who may need urgent resuscitative measures at birth. The bed itself is not the comfortable resting place one might find at home but a high, narrow, industrial model with stirrups to which the woman's legs may be strapped and poles for hanging intravenous lines. The bed is moveable and its shape can change to assist the woman to sit up or lie down, a feature that implies a passivity and inability to control her own movement that is rarely seen in laboring women who are un-medicated. The linen consists of white sheets and pillows without decoration or suggestion of comfort or coziness. Figure 9.1b reveals the prominence of the operating room light positioned over

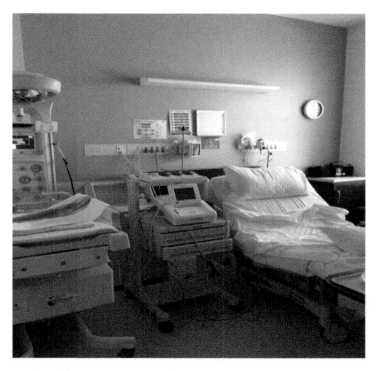

FIGURE 9.1A New South Wales (Australia) Hospital Birth Room

Source: Personal photograph M. Foureur 2016

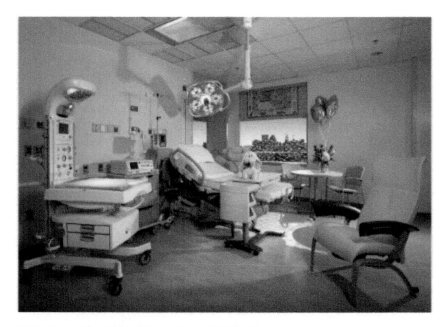

FIGURE 9.1B The Hybrid Space: Hospital Birth Room

Source: With permission from Johns Hopkins Medicine – John Hopkins Birthing Center, USA

the bed to clearly illuminate whatever is happening to the person on the bed. Each object implies its use for something to be done to the woman's body during the process of labor or birth, or to her baby. The narrative is that birth here is a risky event but every risk can be managed with the array of equipment displayed, a narrative that some women find comforting, but most find fearful.

Sanctuary

Figures 9.2a and 9.2b are of a typical modern birth center with an entirely different narrative. Here the prominent feature is a large birth pool/bath for water immersion during labor to aid relaxation and pain relief and potentially water birth. The bath is deep and wide to ensure the woman's pelvis can be completely immersed if the baby is born under water. The wide bed is of a low domestic design and covered with domestic bedding suggesting home-like rest and comfort. Infant resuscitation equipment is contained within the bank of timber cupboards and remains out of sight unless needed. There is no overhead operating room light. At night, the lighting is low and soft suggesting calmness and intimacy. This room design has been described as a sanctuary and meets women's expressed desire for private rooms that have a spa-like aesthetic that suggests they will be treated with respect and gentleness and their bodies will be touched with care.[15]

What impact these differently designed rooms and artifacts have on women's experience and behavior and subsequent birth outcomes is beginning to be explored.[16] One theoretical explanation is that differently designed spaces for birth

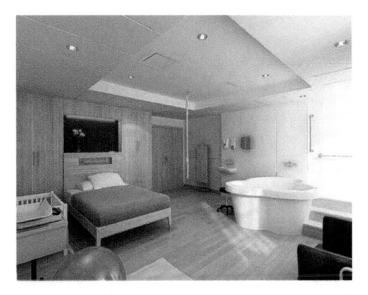

FIGURE 9.2A   Cossham Birth Centre, North Bristol, UK, Day Scene (Google Images, 2016)

Source: With permission from North Bristol NHS Trust

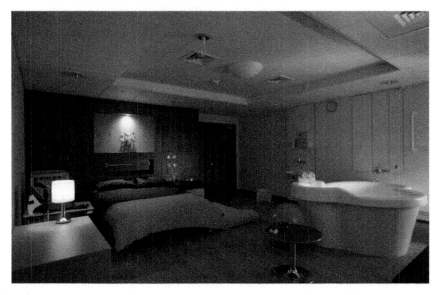

FIGURE 9.2B   Cossham Birth Centre, North Bristol, UK, Night Scene (Google Images, 2016)

Source: With permission from North Bristol NHS Trust

and the artifacts found within may have a significant impact on the neurophysiology of laboring and birthing women.[17] In the next section we explore this idea further.

The Neurophysiology of Mammalian Birth

All mammals share many aspects of the neurophysiology of birth. One shared principle is the need for the birth environment to be experienced as safe-enough for labor and birth to unfold—spaces that are protected, private or hidden away from the eyes of others who may wish to harm the vulnerable mother (at least in the competitive animal world) or her even more vulnerable newborn.[18]

Research in this area has convincingly demonstrated the impact of disrupting this fundamental need for ensuring safe birth environments. Advances in neuroscience have established the role of the brain and "the way a person perceives and orientates themselves in unfamiliar places. . . [establishing how] the environment impacts on cognition, problem solving, pain tolerance and mood".[19,20] A growing number of scientists have begun to examine what has been termed the 'peripartal neurohormonal scenery of the brain' of the mother, her unborn infant and newborn and its role in maternal-infant attachment.[21] These studies reveal a complex interplay of emotion-based neurohormones that orchestrate the physiological process of human reproduction leading to mothering behaviors that ensure the survival of the infant.

Studies of the neuro-hormone oxytocin, which is the main driver of uterine contractions leading to birth (amongst many other complex functions), have revealed its production can be disrupted, slowed or stopped altogether by exposing the laboring female to experiences that are perceived as fearful.[22] This may be as overt as making loud noises or turning on bright lights or roughly handling the mother, or may be as subtle as the rising of the sun that heralds daylight and the possibility that the hidden birth space may be exposed.[23] While laboring women are considered to have more highly developed thought processes than other mammals, it is apparent from correlational research that similar processes can also disrupt the neurohormonal responses of human mammals during labor.[24]

The concept of the "Fear Cascade" describes neurohormonal responses women may have to birth spaces that may be overtly or covertly considered to be unsafe or fear-inducing.[25,26] Decades of research tell us that fear stimulates the brain to produce catecholamines which are brain-based hormones that can alter our physiology and behavior. For example, when the catecholamine adrenaline/epinephrine is secreted in response to experiencing fear, blood is diverted away from the trunk of the body and towards primitive parts of the brain and to the muscles of the arms and legs (to run away, or stand and fight or to maintain stillness and appear immobile, as if dead)—this is the well-known, fight, flight or freeze response.[27] During labor this reaction can cause labor to become irregular, slow down or stop altogether, as adrenaline has a particular inhibiting impact on the release of oxytocin. This is an adaptive response to cues of danger so that the mother can move to a safer place to give birth. Diverting blood to the extremities may also restrict blood supply to the placenta and thereby disrupt the oxygenation of the baby, triggering acidosis in a vulnerable fetus. Once labor has begun, these physiological processes are reflected in the two main reasons for all intervention in childbirth: uterine inertia (the slowing or stopping of uterine contractions) and fetal distress.

The experience of "fear" may not be a conscious response to overt cues, but may occur unconsciously when stimulated by more covert cues from the environment that the eyes may not directly see but that the brain perceives, through its many senses. For example, subtle smells may trigger memories of unpleasant experiences; symbols may trigger negative thoughts or associations; different kinds of light stimulate a range of brain-based bodily functions and behaviors; and surveillance activates the amygdala deep within the limbic system of the brain to translate emotions into actions.[28]

What is increasingly apparent is that the design of many current institutional birth spaces triggers both overt and covert fear responses in laboring women that disrupt the normal neurohormonal or brain-based hormonal control of childbirth. As one woman said:

> I think the message of the hospital at the moment is, "We'll do it for you, you don't need to do anything, just leave it with us, you haven't got very far in the set amount of time we have said, therefore lets whisk this baby out". I don't think there is an acknowledgement that it is a really important part of

the process for women to give birth. Having all that equipment there sends a message—something could go wrong. Therefore, I'm going to need to have that because something is going to go wrong.

(Sheehy)[29]

Adding to the normal stress and pain of labor, constant surveillance of the woman by professional care providers, watching and waiting for something to go wrong, in environments replete with artifacts designed to rescue, is perceived by many as fear-inducing rather than comforting. In recognition of this stress hospitals encourage women to bring one or more supportive companions with them, but providing positive emotional support and encouragement in unfamiliar environments is a challenging task.

Women Need and Want Cooperative, Continuous Supporters

The continuous presence of cooperative, encouraging supporters has been linked to many benefits for the mother and baby.[30] Supporters may be active or passive. The active supporter demonstrates support through eye-to-eye engagement and facial expressions that the woman can easily read and will unconsciously "mirror"[31] or through physical comfort, touch, praise and encouragement. The passive supporter acts as an "observer" with calm patience and by "just being there", which is also valued by women.[32] Anxious, stressed or otherwise uncooperative supporters may create additional feelings of worry or judgment of the woman. Exploring how the built environment facilitates or inhibits the supporters' role provides additional insights into the experiences of women during childbirth.

Supporters Experience an Unbelonging Paradox

A recent Australian video-ethnographic study revealed the designed birth space as having a profound impact on the supporters' experience.[33] Supporters did not feel welcomed or supported in their role by the physical attributes of the space. Video and interview data identified that supporters also need to feel supported in what is an extremely stressful event and revealed their inability to easily negotiate their support role. They experienced what we have identified as an 'unbelonging paradox'—being needed and expected to be present, yet feeling uncertain of what to do and feeling 'in the way' of the birthing woman and her professional carers. The mother of one birthing woman, who served the primary support role in the 'childbirth supporter study', stated:

It just took a while to settle in and just see where are we? Where do we fit in, in this place with everything around there? How do we move around and feel comfortable without being too cautious?

(Florence)[34]

This supporter sought centered, calm focus to attend to her daughter's needs, but experienced equipment everywhere, which made her anxious. She felt as though she might back into it or bump it. The medical equipment was a close, constant presence in both her peripheral vision and her thoughts.

At a neurophysiological level, the supporter who has entered the foreign birth space is likely to feel anxious or even fearful of what is to come, emotions that will be translated into neurohormones that influence behavior. Fear triggers the amygdala that will flood the supporter's brain with adrenalin. This will prevent high level neocortical processing, meaning frightened supporters are less able to problem solve and come up with creative suggestions for how the woman might move or position herself differently in order to feel less discomfort or pain. A level of mental confusion may result that compounds the feeling of 'unbelonging' and not knowing what to do.

Providing Support for the Supporters

Other studies have also shown that childbirth supporters are in need of support themselves.[35] They can be supported by feeling welcome by the care providers, but also by elements of the built space such as intuitive design, comfortable/flexible seating and ample storage for the range of supplies women and their families bring to the birth space to make it more home-like (soft pillows, aromatherapy, comfortable clothing, music). They also can be supported by the presence of easily accessible facilities that address their bodily needs, specifically nourishing food and drink provisions and access to toilet facilities. However, the design of the birth space must also attend to supporters' emotional and physical needs (in human-factors terms, such as protecting their knees and backs), needs that are very similar to those of the woman's professional care providers.

Impact of Currently Designed Spaces on the Woman's Professional Care Providers

Arguably, if the space works well for women and their supporters, it will also be an optimal working environment for the woman's professional care providers who are predominantly midwives and nurse/midwives. Existing research shows that midwives are affected by the spaces and places within which they work and, importantly, studies reveal that they change their practices depending on the environment.[36,37]

A fundamental aspect of the midwives' role in birth is "the initiation and facilitation of trusting social relationships and the provision of emotionally sensitive care".[38] A key mediator of human social and emotional behavior is the neuropeptide oxytocin, which was explored earlier in this chapter. Research examining midwives' reactions to differently designed birth spaces reveal themes that reflect the same emotional and therefore neurophysiological responses to the spaces as experienced by women and their supporters. Midwives' primary goal is to support women to experience a straightforward birth but studies have revealed this is difficult to do in a biomedical birth space where the narrative is one of risk and where constant surveillance is the goal supported in design characteristics.[39] With no support for their professional, psychological or social needs, the birth environment is experienced as stressful for midwives, which generates negative feelings towards the space and their professional and emotional work with women.

In an interview study with 11 midwives working in two differently designed maternity hospitals in Australia, several themes emerged reflecting poor design with inflexible and impractical layouts that were at odds with the professional role of midwives.[40] Themes included "finding a space amongst congestion and clutter; trying to work underwater; creating ambiance in a clinical space and being ill-equipped for flexible practice".[41] Rooms quickly became crowded and cluttered with objects soon after the woman entered since there was inadequate storage for equipment and the woman's belongings. The typical prominent position of the bed in the center of the room was a key component of this inflexibility as reported by one of the midwives:

> Well there isn't anywhere to move it (the bed) out of the way because then you're blocking off some other thing you might need all of a sudden. Everything has got a spot and so if you move the bed over here you've blocked off the oxygen or you've blocked off the sink—it's not flexible. That's how it is and it is very difficult.
>
> *(Annie)*[42]

Surprisingly, there was also no space to accommodate the midwife in the room in which she worked:

> There isn't anywhere for us (to sit) so its almost like you're not meant to (sit down). If you feel you need a break, I would go out to the nurses' station (central desk) because there's not really anywhere in the room that you can go off into a little corner.
>
> *(Annie)*[43]

The midwives frequently supported women who were laboring in either the shower or bath, since there are many documented benefits of water immersion during labor and birth. They found themselves literally 'trying to work underwater'. However, supporting and monitoring women in poorly designed baths caused the midwives considerable discomfort:

> Because of the height of the bath I can't sit down because I can't see. So I'm standing, leaning on my knees as a lever on the bath, leaning over, holding the torch with my left hand, holding the mirror with my right—it hurts. I've got a really sore back.
>
> *(Lisa)*[44]

Midwives reported feeling embarrassed by the inflexibility of the spaces and the poorly designed equipment with which they were forced to work. This resulted in making excuses to the women and their families and trying to cover up or minimize the clumsiness and inadequacies of the environment and its artifacts.

Towards Salutogenic Design for Birth

Salutogenic design for birth requires much more than providing a restful 'ambiance' in the birth space or even simply adding nature views.[45] It requires a narrative that understands childbirth as a complex, neurophysiological process that is, for the most part, not under conscious control. Childbirth is also a social process embedded within a culture and the political and institutional priorities of its time. Both neurophysiological and social perspectives will influence the architect and designer, and the users of the spaces we create. Salutogenic design for birth requires a finely nuanced understanding that every created and curated space is invested with meaning and value and non-verbally proscribes how the space can be used. For straightforward birth to unfold, the environment needs to consider design issues for all users of the space, beginning with meeting the woman's needs for her neurophysiology to remain undisturbed, as paramount.

Salutogenic design elements may include: curved rather than straight lines and sharp angles in walls, ceilings, fixtures and equipment;[46] enveloping nooks as well as open spaces for active movement at different phases of labor;[47] options for water immersion including a deep bath/pool;[48] and no direct line of sight to the spaces where the woman might locate herself so that her privacy is protected at all times.

We propose that the inclusion of more women-centric equipment and 'everyday' design features, as opposed to the current over-abundance of visible medical-surveillance equipment, will also benefit the movement towards normalizing birth, with salutogenically designed birth spaces. Examples of women-centric equipment that the woman may use include: leaning mantels or pull-ropes, plentiful 'yoga'-balls, padded mats for kneeling and beanbags. These are all easy software elements that can be included within the interior design of birth units and can support both the woman and her active supporter.

From a 'hardware' perspective, the design of the birth room should include a floor plan layout with a family alcove—a small space near a window or the entryway to the room, allowing for passive supporters to have access to privacy, while still being together.[49] Importantly, design features that facilitate both space-definition and personal control are an overarching recommendation for the improved design of birth units. Incorporating lighting, temperature, audio and privacy controls that are easy to use (such as adjustable lighting, explicit permission to adjust the climate and audio) will provide increased sense of personal control.

The list of design ideas is long and this chapter can only serve to bring to the architect and designer's attention that there is a need for well-informed salutogenic design for birth. Further resources are available, some in development and others well validated[50] (see the Birth Unit Design Spatial Evaluation Tool—BUDSET, available from www.uts.edu.au/sites/default/files/budset.pdf). Research in this area is ongoing.

Conclusion

No space or place is neutrally constructed.[51,52] Modern imaging technologies and knowledge of neuroendocrinology have enabled us to gain valuable insight into how emotions are used by the limbic system of the brain to constantly monitor the environment to check for danger in order to keep us safe. This system is powerfully in evidence during human reproduction and this chapter has explored how the designed birth space can disrupt neurophysiological birth processes by stimulating the senses to perceive danger and threat. Salutogenic design for birth is not only aimed at reducing anxiety but is primarily focused on negentropic or order-promoting forces that celebrate life-giving. Subsequently, we have provided signposts for the architect and designer wishing to create a salutogenic design for birth. It is not hyperbole to suggest that the future of humanity depends on it.

References

1 Hannah G. Dahlen, Holly P. Kennedy, Cindy M. Anderson, Aleeca F. Bell, Ashley Clark, Maralyn Foureur, Joyce E. Ohm, Amanda M. Shearman, Jacquelyn Y. Taylor, Michelle L. Wright, and Soo Downe, "The EPIIC Hypothesis: Intrapartum Effects on the Neonatal Epigenome and Consequent Health Outcomes," *Medical Hypotheses* 80, no. 5 (2013): 656–662.
2 Aaron Antonovsky, *Health, Stress, and Coping* (San Francisco, CA: Jossey-Bass Publishers, 1985).
3 Jan Golembiewski, "Salutogenic Architecture in Health Care Settings," in *Handbook of Salutogenics: Past, Present and Future*, eds. Maurice B. Mittelmark, Shifra Sagy, Monica Eriksson, Georg Bauer, Jürgen M. Pelikan, Bengt Lindström, and Geir Arild Espnes (New York: Springer, 2016): 267-276.
4 Alan Dilani, "The Beneficial Health Outcomes of Salutogenic Design," *Design & Health Scientific Review* 28 (2015): 18–35.
5 Ank de Jonge, Birgit Y. van der Goes, Anita C. J. Ravelli, Marianne P. Amelink-Verburg, Ben W. Mol, Jan G. Nijhuis, J. Bennebroek Gravenhorst, and Simone E. Buitendijk, "Perinatal Mortality and Morbidity in a Nationwide Cohort of 529, 688 Low-Risk Planned Home and Hospital Births," *BJOG: An International Journal of Obstetrics & Gynaecology* 116, no. 9 (2009): 1177–1184.
6 Doris Haire, "Cultural Warping of Childbirth," *International Childbirth Education Association News* 11, no. 1 (1972): 5–35.
7 Mary Newburn and Debbie Singh, *Are Women Getting the Birth Environment They Need: Report of a National Survey of Women's Experiences* (London: National Childbirth Trust, 2005).
8 Birthplace in England Collaborative Group, "Perinatal and Maternal Outcomes by Planned Place of Birth for Healthy Women With Low Risk Pregnancies: The Birthplace in England National Prospective Cohort Study," *BMJ* 343, no. 7840 (2011): d7400.
9 Eileen K. Hutton, Adriana Cappelletti, Angela H. Reitsma, Julia Simioni, Jordyn Horne, Caroline McGregor, and Rashid J. Ahmed, "Outcomes Associated With Planned Place of Birth Among Women With Low-Risk Pregnancies," *CMAJ: Canadian Medical Association Journal = Journal De L'association Medicale Canadienne* 188, no. 5 (2015): E80–E90.
10 Jonge, "Perinatal Mortality."

11 Billie Hunter, Marie Berg, Ingela Lundgren, Ólöf Ásta Ólafsdóttir, and Mavis Kirkham, "Relationships: The Hidden Threads in the Tapestry of Maternity Care," *Midwifery* 24, no. 2 (2008): 132–137.

12 Jane Sandall, Hora Soltani, Simon Gates, Andrew Shennan, and Declan Devane, "Midwife-Led Continuity Models Versus Other Models of Care for Childbearing Women," *Cochrane Pregnancy and Childbirth Group; Cochrane Database of Systematic Reviews* (2016).

13 Ivy Lynn Bourgeault, Rebecca Sutherns, Margaret MacDonald, and Jacquelyne Luce, "Problematising Public and Private Work Spaces: Midwives' Work in Hospitals and in Homes," *Midwifery* 28, no. 5 (2012): 582–590.

14 Bethan Townsend, Jennifer Fenwick, Val Thomson, and Maralyn Foureur, "The Birth Bed: A Qualitative Study on the Views of Midwives Regarding the Use of the Bed in the Birth Space," *Women and Birth* 29 (2015): 80–84.

15 Annabel Sheehy, Maralyn Foureur, Christine Catling-Paull, and Caroline S. E. Homer, "Examining the Content Validity of the Birthing Unit Design Spatial Evaluation Tool Within a Woman-Centered Framework," *The Journal of Midwifery & Women's Health* 56, no. 5 (2011): 494–502.

16 Maree Stenglin and Maralyn Foureur, "Designing Out the Fear Cascade to Increase the Likelihood of Normal Birth," *Midwifery* 29, no. 8 (May 2013): 819–825.

17 Maralyn Foureur, Deborah L. Davis, Jennifer Fenwick, Nicky Leap, Rick Iedema, Ian F. Forbes, and Caroline S. E. Homer, "The Relationship Between Birth Unit Design and Safe, Satisfying Birth: Developing a Hypothetical Model," *Midwifery* 26, no. 5 (2010): 520–525.

18 Stenglin, "Fear Cascade."

19 Carolyn Hastie, "The Birthing Environment: A Sustainable Approach," in *Sustainability, Midwifery and Birth*, eds. L. Davies, R. Daellenbach, and M. Kensington (Abingdon, Oxon: Routledge, 2011), 103, 101–114.

20 Esther M. Sternberg and Matthew A. Wilson, "Neuroscience and Architecture: Seeking Common Ground," *Cell* 127, no. 2 (2006): 239–242.

21 Ibone Olza-Fernández, Miguel Angel Marín Gabriel, Alfonso Gil-Sanchez, Luis M. Garcia-Segura, and Maria Angeles Arevalo, "Neuroendocrinology of Childbirth and Mother—Child Attachment: The Basis of an Etiopathogenic Model of Perinatal Neuro-biological Disorders," *Frontiers in Neuroendocrinology* 35, no. 4 (2014): 459–472.

22 Jerónima M. A. Teixeira, Nicholas M. Fisk, and Vivette Glover, "Association Between Maternal Anxiety in Pregnancy and Increased Uterine Artery Resistance Index: Cohort Based Study," *BMJ* 318, no. 7177 (1999): 153–157.

23 Martin Dicken, Erica K. Gee, Chris W. Rogers, and I. G. Joe Mayhew, "Gestation Length and Occurrence of Daytime Foaling of Standardbred Mares on Two Stud Farms in New Zealand," *New Zealand Veterinary Journal* 60, no. 1 (2012): 42–46.

24 Cornelius Naaktgeboren, "The Biology of Childbirth," in *Effective Care in Pregnancy and Childbirth*, eds. Iain Chalmers, Murray W. Enkin, and Mark J. Keirse (Oxford: Oxford University Press, 1989), 795–804.

25 Kathleen Fahy, Maralyn Foureur, and Carolyn Hastie, eds. *Birth Territory and Midwifery Guardianship: Theory for Practice, Education and Research* (Oxford, UK: Elsevier, 2008).

26 Stenglin, "Fear Cascade."

27 Norman B. Schmidt, J. Anthony Richey, Michael J. Zvolensky, and Jon K. Maner, "Exploring Human Freeze Responses to a Threat Stressor," *Journal of Behavior Therapy and Experimental Psychiatry* 39, no. 3 (2008): 292–304.

28 Stenglin, "Fear Cascade."

29 Sheehy, "Content Validity," 498.

30 Ellen D. Hodnett, Simon Gates, G. Justus Hofmeyr, and Carol Sakala, "Continuous Support for Women During Childbirth," Cochrane Database of Systematic Reviews 2012, Issue 10. Art. No.: CD003766. DOI: 10.1002/14651858.CD003766.pub4.

31 Stephen Porges, *The Polyvagal Theory: Neurophysiological Foundations of Emotions, Attachment, Communication, Self-Regulation* (New York: W.W. Norton and Co Ltd, 2011).

32 Hanna-Leena Melender, "What Constitutes a Good Childbirth? A Qualitative Study of Pregnant Finnish Women," *Journal of Midwifery & Women's Health* 51, no. 5 (2006): 331–339.

33 J. Davis Harte, Athena Sheehan, Susan C. Stewart, and Maralyn Foureur, "Childbirth Supporters' Experiences in a Built Hospital Birth Environment: Exploring Inhibiting and Facilitating Factors," *HERD: Health Environments Research & Design Journal* 9, no. 3 (2016): 135–161.

34 Harte, "Supporters' Experiences," 144.

35 Susan Chandler and Peggy Ann Field, "Becoming a Father: First-Time Fathers' Experience of Labor and Delivery," *Journal of Nurse-Midwifery* 42, no. 1 (1997): 17–24.

36 Deborah Davis and Kim Walker, "The Corporeal, the Social and Space/Place: Exploring Intersections From a Midwifery Perspective in New Zealand," *Gender, Place and Culture* 17, no. 3 (2010): 377–391.

37 Athena Hammond, Maralyn Foureur, and Caroline S. E. Homer, "The Hardware and Software Implications of Hospital Birth Room Design: A Midwifery Perspective," *Midwifery* 30, no. 7 (2014): 825–830.

38 Athena Hammond, Maralyn Foureur, Caroline S. E. Homer, and Deborah L. Davis, "Space, Place and the Midwife: Exploring the Relationship Between the Birth Environment, Neurobiology and Midwifery Practice," *Women and Birth* 26, no. 4 (2013): 277.

39 Athena Hammond, Caroline S. E. Homer, and Maralyn Foureur, "Messages From Space: An Exploration of the Relationship Between Hospital Birth Environments and Midwifery Practice," *HERD: Health Environments Research & Design Journal* 7, no. 4 (2014): 81–95.

40 Ibid.

41 Hammond, "Hardware and Software," 826.

42 Ibid.

43 Ibid., 827.

44 Ibid.

45 Roger S. Ulrich, Craig Zimring, Xuemei Zhu, Jennifer DuBose, Hyun-Bo Seo, Young-Seon Choi, Xiaobo Quan, and Anjali Joseph, "A Review of the Research Literature on Evidence-Based Healthcare Design," *The Health Environments Research & Design Journal* 1, no. 3 (2008): 61–125.

46 Letizia Palumbo, Nicole Ruta, and Marco Bertamini. "Comparing Angular and Curved Shapes in Terms of Implicit Associations and Approach/Avoidance Responses," *PloS One* 10, no. 10 (2015): e0140043.

47 Letizia Palumbo et al., "Comparing Angular and Curved Shapes."

48 Stenglin, "Fear Cascade."

49 Robyn M. Maude and Maralyn J. Foureur, "It's Beyond Water: Stories of Women's Experience of Using Water for Labour and Birth," *Women and Birth* 20, no. 1 (2007): 17–24.

50 Sheehy, "Content Validity."

51 Hammond, "Space, Place and Midwife."

52 Hammond, "Messages."

10

HEALTHY SCHOOLS, HEALTHY LIFESTYLES: LITERATURE REVIEW

*Carole Després, Andrée-Anne Larivière-Lajoie,
Sandrine Tremblay-Lemieux, Marianne Legault,
and Denise Piché*

Introduction: Problem Statement

In Quebec, Canada, 85 percent of the province's 2,158 primary schools were built before 1970, two-thirds between 1950 and 1970 to serve the baby boom.[1] Most of these buildings have reached the end of their first life cycle, estimated as 50 years in architecture. The obsolescence of the school estate is regularly decried in the media. Its updating has been identified as a priority by Quebec's government, which will be investing over $8,9B to renovate and expand the elementary and secondary school facilities until 2026. This major operation represents a unique opportunity to inform designers with the best scientific and practiced-based evidences. Beyond construction or green-building considerations, architectural interventions should be guided to better serve the educational mission and also to support children's health and well-being. Quebec's Public Health Agency (INSPQ) recently targeted the renovation of school infrastructure as a priority strategy to encourage the adoption of healthy lifestyles among youth.[2] In Quebec, the pedagogical reforms carried out since 1964 had little impact on the facilities (except for the addition of gymnasiums, kindergarten classes or information technologies). However, the daily life of children has considerably evolved since the schools were first built. While the baby boomers walked to school and went home or to a family member's house for lunch, the great majority of their grandchildren go to and from school in a car or a bus and has lunch there. With 85.7 percent of women with children aged 5 to 11 working outside the home in 2009,[3] the number of pupils using in-school childcare services increased by about 30-fold since its introduction in 1979.[4] In 2010, children spent an average of 60 percent more time at school than they did in 1950.[5] Increased hours of informal education raise questions about the division of work between teachers and educators,[6] as well as about fatigue and stress. Sedentary behaviors[7] and poor nutrition[8] have also been associated with higher obesity risks, a concern in Canada where the number of overweight children has literally doubled since 1978 and now affects 31 percent of children aged 5 to 11.[9] Finally, school environments have become more complex, serving pupils with special needs, such as ADHD, autism, physical limitations, or else, with different cultural and socioeconomic backgrounds. Non-teaching professionals such as speech therapists or social workers have joined the staff to accompany the students. In sum, over the years, schools have become not only a place for instruction, but a genuine living space where teachers, professionals and educators play a complementary role in the education, health and well-being of the children. This being said, the school estate is out of step with this reality. How can researcher-designers participate in the renovation of schools and contribute to adapting it to its expanded mission?

Theoretical and Methodological Strategy

To inform the renovation of the schools in a relatively limited timeframe, it is essential to make intelligent use of the best knowledge available to support decision-making. This requires combining *scientific evidences* from different disciplinary horizons with local information on local organizational and material contexts or *practice-based evidences*. The former is the outcome of research that is peer-reviewed before publication, in scientific journals for the most part; the latter, of case studies which generally remain unpublished. These two forms of knowledge need to be cross-fertilized and translated into user-friendly decision-aid tools, accessible to designers and to the various parties involved in the decision process. An important step is to search databases for scientific evidences. The next section presents the literature review conducted in three consecutive steps between 2014 and 2016. After applying selected exclusion criteria to the 827 records initially identified, we were left with ten literature reviews and 61 articles reporting on original studies, all published between 2009 and 2016 (see Figure 10.1).

About 70 percent of the selected articles report on studies conducted in Anglo-Saxon countries (U.S. [30], United Kingdom [9], Australia [7], New Zealand [4], Canada [2]); the others were from Scandinavian (4) or other European countries (7), the Middle East (3) and Brazil (2). Three additional studies were conducted simultaneously in two or more countries, associating Canada and Australia, Belgium and Germany or Italy and the U.S. Sixty-four percent of articles are signed by authors trained in the same field of research and knowledge, the great majority in health-related disciplines such as nutrition, ergonomics, medicine, etc. (31), the others in education (4), sciences and engineering (3), human and social sciences (3) and administration and management (2). Two studies were led by researchers in architecture or design only. In addition, 26 articles are the outcome of collaborations between two or more of the above research fields, among which 11 associating architecture, design or planning with health, geography, education, social sciences or engineering. Half of the methodologies included objective measures of health or healthy behaviors, namely body measures and calculated BMI, heart rate telemetry, body motion; 11 studies included a validated inventory and observation protocol

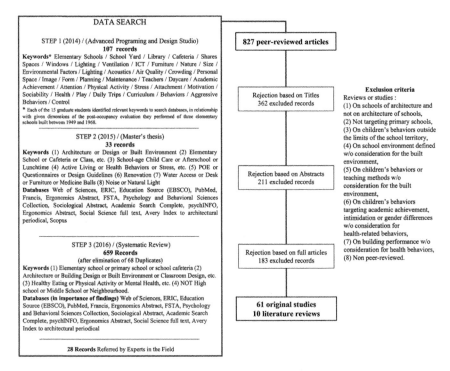

FIGURE 10.1 Search Process for the Literature Review on the Contribution of the Built Environment to Healthy Schools and Lifestyles

Source: Sandrine Tremblay-Lemieux

(e.g., SOPLAY). Half of the studies surveyed teachers, pupils, directors or parents, using self-reported questionnaires (30), in-person or phone interviews (8) or focus groups (4). Subjective health evaluations were obtained from self-reported symptoms of stress, headaches and asthma. In schoolyards, objective measures of the built environment consisted in measuring areas, checking for the presence of equipment and counting elements (6); in classrooms, levels of noise, room temperature, etc., were measured (6), as well as furniture height, depth and other characteristics (6).

Results

Schoolyards

Over half of the reviewed articles (32 articles and six literature reviews) focused on elementary schoolyards or playgrounds. In Canada and Australia, at least 25 percent of children's daily school time is estimated to be spent there.[10] The *improvement or redesign* of schoolyards has been repeatedly associated with an increase in students' use and activity levels.[11-15] The transformations consisted of adding play equipment, paved or green areas,[16] fences, shading devices, gardens and artwork,[11] color ground markings and refurbishment.[15,16] A positive association was repeatedly found in 12 articles between the presence, quantity and/or quality of *play equipment* and levels of physical activity.[17-28] Equipment is alternately understood as grass, sand or paved areas for play, sports fields (dedicated or line-marked), jogging tracks and pools, structures (climbing frames/walls, nets, fort platforms, bars and bridges), swings and stands, mobile devices (balls, tools, rocks, etc.). Only one study did not find any significant association between levels of physical activity and the number of outdoor facilities, as reported by students and principals.[29]

Lack of space can act as a barrier to body motion.[30] The size of the schoolyard has been positively associated with outdoor recreation time[31] and levels of physical activity,[32] although self-reported activities did not allow for such conclusions.[33] It is rather the landscape diversity that seems to stimulate children's play.[14,30] Observations of schoolyards' *paved areas* show that they are the most used places,[19] but also that they generate sedentary play.[10] A literature review by Escalante, et al.[34] identified *playgrounds marking* as a low-cost solution to encourage higher levels of physical activity, as confirmed in four studies.[15,16,22,35] Yildirim, et al.[36] in Australia, and Black, et al.[19] in the U.S. respectively found no association or a reversed relationship between higher levels of physical activity and the availability of line markings. Because little information is provided on the types of marking that range from simple lines delimiting sports fields to colorful and diversified playground markings (castles, clock faces, mazes, ladders, animals, hopscotch), it is somewhat hard to make sense of the evidences. Two studies suggest that the activity levels are higher in free games compared to those organized.[10,37]

Brittin et al.'s review[12] also suggests that *green spaces* contribute to increasing physical activity among children, as confirmed by a Canadian-Australian research[10] and another Australian one.[38] It was also associated with lower levels of stress in two studies of multiple schools in the U.S.[39] and in Spain.[40] Green spaces were where more pupils gather, specifically girls, although grassy berms with trees were found to favor sedentary behaviors.[10] The presence of deciduous or coniferous trees, large and small, was positively correlated with outdoor recreation time,[31] with children reporting areas with trees, bushes and benches as their most appreciated places.[41] *Shady areas* were also associated with higher levels of physical activity,[10] with shade on play equipment where needed increasing the use of schoolyards.[11,42] Another Australian study by Martin et al.[43] reports otherwise, with more active children on less shady grass surfaces. Three literature reviews discuss the limitations of these findings in terms of the season in which the studies were conducted. Climate conditions (temperature, sun, wind, rain, snow, etc.) may indeed help interpret diverging scientific evidences, influencing the areas of a schoolyard that are being used or preferred by children throughout the year.

The presence of a *vegetable garden* was associated with moderate physical activity.[10,30,44] Three literature reviews conclude that a vegetable garden contributes to young people learning how to feed themselves more properly,[45,46] by providing namely holistic food, nutrition education, tasting and cooking opportunities.[47]

Frerichs et al.[45] reports that among 21 studies assessing school garden programs in the U.S., the UK and Australia, six identified positive dietary behavior outcomes and nine dietary-related psychosocial outcomes.

Classrooms

Nineteen records take the classroom as the main unit of analysis. A first subgroup is concerned by environmental factors and how they impact children's health and comfort (one literature review and six original studies). In their literature review, Zomorodian et al.[48] stress that low air quality and thermal discomfort lead to dangerous situations for health due to the high density of students occupying the same room or the hypersensitivity of children to upper temperatures. Overheating is often caused by solar gains and unsuited ventilation (such as closed windows to keep away outdoor noises). Children were found to have a different metabolic rate compared to adults; a study in the UK shows that pupils get warmer faster and remain comfortable longer in lower temperatures in a classroom than established standards for adults.[49] Poor air quality, influenced by ambient temperature and ventilation, was associated with children's nasal congestion and asthma in the UK[50] and in Finland.[51] The Finnish study of 297 schools suggests that not only poor air quality but also high noise levels are the most often reported factors associated with a stuffy nose, fatigue and headaches.[51] High noise levels were also linked to stress,[52] as measured on children of two Swedish classes by cortisol variation, a hormone released in response to stress, as well as self-reported symptoms of fatigue and headaches. In a large Scottish survey, the intensity of light levels in classrooms was also found to affect space utilization; pupils' mood and levels of activity were higher in sunny rooms compared to shaded ones.[53] De Giuli et al.[54] conclude that if children react actively to environmental discomfort (objectively measured temperature, relative humidity, illuminance, air velocity, air quality and noise levels), they have little control over their environment.

The second subgroup of 12 studies addressed the classroom furniture, its placement, type and ergonomics in relationship to student's physical comfort or energy expenditure. Six of them, conducted in Brazil, Greece, India, Portugal and Saudi Arabia, evaluated class furniture in terms of its adaptation to children's bodies. Furniture was generally unfitted, being too deep or too high for the majority of children,[55,56] and did not allow for different body postures,[57] generating work, writing or seating discomfort. Headaches were the most reported complaint, followed by leg, shoulder, hand and neck discomforts.[58] Ramadan[59] achieved similar conclusions after measuring six combinations of desks and chairs. Testing the inclination of different tables or chairs, Gonçalves and Arezes[60] found that tilted desk tops were the most appreciated by children and contributed in reducing trunk and neck tensions. Six additional studies tested classroom alternative desk and chair solutions to reduce sitting time and increase energy expenditure. Cardon et al.[61] found that standing desks increase daily caloric expenditure compared to traditional sitting, as measured with accelerometers in two classes in Germany and Belgium.

In New Zealand, comparing traditional sitting to standing stations and alternate sitting (Swiss balls, beanbags, benches and mat space), Aminian et al.[62] measured a significant one-hour daily increase in standing. More specifically, Benden et al.[63,64] and Blake et al.[65] found that students using alternate furniture significantly burned more calories. Blake et al.[65] even reported that by the fourth week of the intervention, over two-thirds of the pupils stop using their stool, removing it from their workstations and preferring to stand up. Comparing children's time spent sitting, standing and walking, as well as step counts, sit-to-stand transitions and musculoskeletal discomfort, with traditional desks and standing workstations, the same group of researchers found that it is the variations in body positions that led to higher-calorie expenses.[66] Comparing these two sitting arrangements, with an "activity-permissive environment" (standing desks, mobile white boards, wireless laptop computers, and portable video display units), Americans Lanningham-Foster, et al.[67] reported that physical activity using standing desk and traditional desk classrooms did not show significant differences, while it was increased by 53 percent in the activity-permissive environment.

Gymnasiums, Motor Rooms and Lunch Areas

When it comes to healthy lifestyles with regards to active living and good nutrition, indoor sports facilities as well as lunch areas are important components to look at, even more so for renovating a school estate built before physical education became mandatory and school daycare established. However, scientific evidences on these spaces come from a much less fertile ground. Four relevant literature reviews discuss these components in relationship with obesity,[68] physical activity[12,69] and healthy eating;[45] In addition, four original studies were also identified.

Inside the school, gymnasiums are traditional places for performing physical activity. Beyond consideration for their acoustics reported as not optimal because of noisy mechanics[70] and their strategic location within the buildings contributing to increasing the time dedicated to physical activity,[71,72] no studies investigated innovating features or uses. In a review of child development theories, Rigolon and Alloway[73] argue that because students physically develop at various rates during elementary school years, multiple types of spaces dedicated to sports should be offered. In Minnesota (U.S.), McCrady-Spitzer et al.[74] monitored the contribution of a "motor room" (ladder, a balance beam, hopscotch, monkey bars and gymnastic mats) to physical activity (accelerometers) and learning (early literacy skills tests). Used by children 30–40 minutes a day over a 28-week period, it increased daily physical activity by 46 percent, with no impact on their literacy.

Lunch areas in schools have been studied in their contribution to healthy nutrition. In their literature review, Frerichs et al.[45] identified several barriers that can infringe the implementation of healthy eating programs: too short meal time (for serving long waiting lines and affecting food choice), insufficient and crowded dining areas and cafeterias (hindering socialization behaviors) and lack of water access (encouraging drinking sugar-sweetened beverages). Four studies associated the shortage of space to the obligation for school administrations to shorten lunch time, which indirectly made it difficult to integrate healthy eating habits, the necessity to eat more rapidly influencing the food choice.[75-77] Longer lunch periods were even associated with a diminution of obesity risks.[78] During focus groups in Australia, parents identified the lack of time for eating and the lack of refrigeration equipment as the main barriers preventing healthy choices for the lunch box, in terms of types and amount of food.[75] A study of the lunch environments in UK schools concludes that lunch areas are operated as "refueling stations" rather than places where children could learn to enjoy nutritious meals, together with table and social skills.[77] Indeed, issues reported by mid-day supervisors, catering staff and teachers suggest that the end-goal was to get each child fed and moved into the playground so that their place could be cleared away. The availability of vegetables and water was identified as having positive impacts on healthy eating habits in two studies. The addition of a salad bar in the cafeteria of three Los Angeles (U.S.) schools increased the daily food and vegetable consumption of children using the facilities by 84 percent over two months,[79] while the installation of a first water fountain significantly increased the consumption of water, as measured by flow meters, over a 19-month period.[80]

Discussion: What Have We Learned?

What has this literature review taught us about the usefulness of science to redesign elementary schools? Can the above evidences inform their transformation to support healthier lifestyles? *The answer is yes and no.*

Yes, because this field of research is not only prolific but anchored in rigorous methodologies and in rich protocols. Instrumental measurements, structured observations and self-assessments are often used simultaneously to monitor, before and after, the effectiveness of an intervention in one school, or to compare multiple ones. One also senses the emergence of international studies, with researchers networking across countries as well as sharing protocols and validated instruments. The answer is *no* for three reasons. First, most methodologies target almost exclusively the classrooms. Because schools have become not only a place for formal education but for learning and practicing behaviors associated with healthy lifestyles, research must also invade the eating areas, the childcare services, as well as the locker rooms, the corridors and the hallways. To accommodate this renewed vocation, architects who will be responsible for renovation mandates need to understand the building in its global functioning. Second, too many researchers lack generosity in describing the geographical contexts of their studies, among which the length and specificity of seasons, schools' solar orientation and siting relative to the prevailing winds and weather conditions during measurement, making it difficult to interpret the scientific evidences (including divergent ones) and translate those into design criteria applicable to general contexts.

Third, and importantly, only a small fraction of the 827 studies identified investigate the built environment itself. Indeed, our literature review excluded hundreds of records defining the school strictly in terms of learning or social environment, with a focus on teaching methods or children's behaviors. Even among the reviewed studies, the variables describing the schools' physical components are not always selected or operationalized as designers would. Floor plans are analyzed in only four studies, building construction periods specified in only three, and metric or qualitative data describing building types (configuration, number of stories, spatial organization, length of corridors, floor areas, etc.) practically ignored. Occupation densities such as the ratio of pupils per square meter are rarely mentioned; so are normative space standards used for facility programming. Three studies out of four do not even show pictures of the targeted school(s) (inside or outside). Consequently, the potential contribution of architecture, furniture or equipment on children's health and lifestyles might be underestimated or misinterpreted. Finally, scientific evidences are not enough to inform design; they must be translated into performance criteria and combined with practiced-based knowledge to produce useful and accessible decision-aid tools. Among the ten literature reviews, only two specifically aimed at feeding design guidelines: the one by Frerichs et al.,[45] used by Huang et al.[81] on healthy eating, and the one by Brittin et al.[12] on physical activity, both the work of the same research network. If commendable efforts were also made, led by practicing architects, to gather "practiced-based evidences" (based on post-occupancy evaluations, collaborative programming and/or best practices) in friendly formats, the results rarely rely on scientific evidences and almost exclusively target the improvement of academic learning and achievement.[82]

Conclusion: What Is Next?

The low involvement of designers in this field of studies where health-related researchers dominate is alarming. Of the 71 articles reviewed, two were carried out by architects or designers only, with 11 more by teams that included some. These results suggest that it is time for architects and other designers to engage in scientific practice, as knowledge producers, knowledge translators and knowledge users. It is also time for academia to revise their curricula. At the undergraduate level, students should be taught human behaviors as associated with the built environment, as well as how to use decision-aid tools to inform design. At the graduate level, professional programs should include developing basic skills in research literacy, as well as in interdisciplinary and multi-sectoral collaborations to produce practiced-based knowledge. At post-professional levels, designers should be trained to act as knowledge translators and agents of change, capable of searching for, interpreting and translating scientific evidences into design or performance criteria, as well as organizing and leading collaborative programming and design processes.[83]

In Quebec as elsewhere in the world, the ongoing renovation of postwar schools represents a unique opportunity to adapt these buildings to answer new challenges. The door is open for designers and decision makers to do a better job, with possible benefits for countless children, teachers and educators. Let's make sure science contributes to it.

References

1 Carole Després, Andrée-Anne Larivière-Lajoie, Marianne Legault, Sandrine Tremblay-Lemieux, and Mélanie Watchman, "La Période Du Dîner Dans Les Écoles Primaires Du Québec." In *Progress Report to the AQGS*. Quebec: GIRBa, Laval University, (2015).

2 Yann Le Bodo, Chantal Blouin, Nathalie Dumas, Philippe De Wals, and Johanne Laguë, *Comment Faire Mieux? L'expérience Québécoise En Promotion Des Saines Habitudes De Vie Et En Prévention De L'obésité*. Edited by Institut national en santé publique. Québec: Presses de l'Université Laval, (2016).

3 Ministère de la Famille et des Ainés (MFA), *Un Portrait Statistique Des Familles Au Québec*. Edited by Louise Dallaire, Paul Marchand, and Joanie Migneault, 325–71. Québec, Gouvernement du Québec, (2011).

4 Data provided by the Quebec Association of School Daycares (AQGS), 2015.

5 Conseil Supérieur de l'Éducation (CSE). *Mieux Accueillir Et Éduquer Les Enfants D'âge Préscolaire, Une Triple Question D'accès De Qualité Et De Continuité Des Services, Avis À La Ministre De L'éducation Des Loisirs Et Du Sport*. Québec: Bibliothèque et Archives Nationales du Québec, (2012).

6 Maurice Tardif and Louis Levasseur, *La division du travail éducatif: une perspective nord-américaine*. France: Presses universitaires de France, (2010).

7 Rachel C. Colley, Suzy L. Wong, Didier Garriguet, Ian Janssen, Sarah Connor Gorber, and Mark S. Tremblay, "Activité Physique, Comportement Sédentaire Et Sommeil Chez Les Enfants Au Canada." In *Rapports sur la santé* 23, no. 2. Statistique Canada, (2012): 49-57.

8 Ministère de l'Éducation, des Loisirs et du Sport (MELS), Going the Healthy Route at School. Framework Policy on Healthy Eating and Active Living. Québec, Canada: Gouvernement du Québec, (2007). ISBN 978-2-550-50588-4 (PDF).

9 Karen C. Roberts, Margot Shields, Margaret de Groh, Alfred Aziz, and Jo-Anne Gilbert, "L'embonpoint Et L'obésité Chez Les Enfants Et Les Adolescents." In *Rapports sur la santé* 23 no. 3. Statistique Canada, (2012).

10 Janet E. Dyment, Anne C. Bell, and Adam J. Lucas, "The Relationship between School Ground Design and Intensity of Physical Activity." *Children's Geographies* 7, no. 3 (2009): 261–76.

11 Peter Anthamatten, Lois Brink, Sarah Lampe, Emily Greenwood, Beverly Kingston, and Claudio Nigg, "An Assessment of Schoolyard Renovation Strategies to Encourage Children's Physical Activity." *International Journal of Behavioral Nutrition & Physical Activity* 8, no. 1 (2011): 27–35.

12 Jeri Brittin, Dina Sorensen, Matthew Trowbridge, Karen K. Lee, Dieter Breithecker, Leah Frerichs, and Terry Huang, "Physical Activity Design Guidelines for School Architecture." *Plos One* 10, no. 7 (2015) e0132597. doi:10.1371/journal.pone.0132597.

13 Natali Colabianchi, Audrey E. Kinsella, Claudia J. Coulton, and Shirley M. Moore, "Utilization and Physical Activity Levels at Renovated and Unrenovated School Playgrounds." *Preventive Medicine* 48, no. 2 (2009): 140–3.

14 Flo Harrison and Andrew P. Jones, "A Framework for Understanding School Based Physical Environmental Influences on Childhood Obesity." *Health & Place* 18, no. 3 (2012): 639–48.

15 Nicola D. Ridgers, Gareth Stratton, Stuart Fairclough, and Jos W. R. Twisk, "Long-Term Effects of a Playground Markings and Physical Structures on Children's Recess Physical Activity Levels." *Preventive Medicine* 44, no. 5 (2007): 393–7.

16 Lois A. Brink, Claudio R. Nigg, Sarah M. R. Lampe, Beverly A. Kingston, Andrew L. Mootz, and Willem van Vliet, "Influence of Schoolyard Renovations on Children's Physical Activity." *American Journal of Public Health* 100, no. 9 (2010): 1672–78.

17 Peter Anthamatten, Lois Brink, Beverly Kingston, Eve Kutchman, Sarah Lampe, and Claudio Nigg, "An Assessment of Schoolyard Features and Behavior Patterns in Children's Utilization and Physical Activity." *Journal Physical Active Health* 11, no. 3 (2014): 564–73.

18 Peter Anthamatten, Erin Fiene, Eve Kutchman, Melanie Mainar, Lois Brink, Ray Browning, and Claudio Nigg, "A Microgeographic Analysis of Physical Activity Behavior Within Elementary School Grounds." *American Journal of Health Promotion* 28, no. 6 (2014): 403–12.

19 Ipuna Estavillo Black, Nancy Nivison Menzel, and Timothy J. Bungum, "The Relationship Among Playground Areas and Physical Activity Levels in Children." *Journal of Pediatric Health Care* 29, no. 2 (2015): 156–68.

20 Thayse Natasha Gomes, Fernanda K. dos Santos, Weimo Zhu, Joey Eisenmann, and José A. R. Maia, "Multilevel Analyses of School and Children's Characteristics Associated with Physical Activity." *Journal of School Health* 84, no. 10 (2014): 668–76.

21 Brook E. Harmon, Claudio R. Nigg, Carmonia Long, Katie Amato, Anwar, Eve Kutchman, Peter Anthamatten, Raymond C. Brownong, Lois Brink, and James O. Hill, "Influence of Social Cognitive Theory and Perceived Environment on Levels of Physical Activity." *Psychology of Sport and Exercise* 15, no. 3 (2014): 272–9.

22 Jennifer L. Huberty, Mohammad Siapush, Aaron Beighle, Erin Fuhrmeister, Pedro Silva, and Greg Welk, "A Pilot Study to Increase Physical Activity in Elementary School Children." *Journal of School Health* 81, no. 5 (2011): 251–7.

23 Jennifer L. Huberty, Michael W. Beets, Aaron Beighle, Pedro F. Saint-Maurice, and Greg Welk, "Effects of Ready for Recess, an Environmental Intervention, on Physical Activity in Third- through Sixth-Grade Children." *Journal of Physical Activity & Health* 11, no. 2 (2014): 384–95.

24 Brendon P. Hyndman, Amanda C. Benson, Shahid Ullah, and Amanda Telford, "Children's Enjoyment of Play During School Lunchtime Breaks." *Journal of Physical Activity & Health* 11, (2014): 109–17.

25 Scott T. Leatherdale, "A Cross-Sectional Examination of School Characteristics Associated With Overweight and Obesity Among Grade 1 to 4 Students." *BMC Public Health* 13, (2013): 982. DOI: 10.1186/1471-2458-13-982.

26 Thomas L. McKenzie, Noe C. Crespo, Barbara Baquero, and John P. Elder, "Leisure-Time Physical Activity in Elementary Schools." *Journal of School Health* 80, no. 10 (2010): 470–7.

27 Mohammad Siahpush, Jennifer L. Huberty, and Aaron Beighle, "Does the Effect of a School Recess Intervention on Physical Activity Vary by Gender or Race?" *Journal of Public Health Management and Practice* 18, no. 5 (2012): 416–22.

28 Rachel W. Taylor, Victoria L. Farmer, Sonya L. Cameron, Kim Meredith-Jones, Sheila M. Williams, and Jim I. Mann, "School Playgrounds and Physical Activity Policies as Predictors of School and Home Time Activity." *International Journal of Behavioral Nutrition & Physical Activity* 8 (2011): 1–7.

29 Ellen Haug, Torbjørn Torsheim, James F. Sallis, and Oddrun Samdal, "The Characteristics of the Outdoor School Environment Associated With Physical Activity." *Health Education Research* 25, no. 2 (2010): 248–56.

30 Janet E. Dyment, and Anne C. Bell, "Active by Design: Promoting Physical Activity Through School Ground Greening." *Children's Geographies* 5, no. 4 (2007): 463–77.

31 Kelley L. Arbogast, Brian C. P. Kane, Jeffrey L. Kirwan, and Bradley R. Hertel, "Vegetation and Outdoor Recess Time at Elementary Schools." *Journal of Environmental Psychology* 29, no. 4 (2009): 450–456.

32 Sara D'Haese, Delfien Van Dyck, Ilse De Bourdeaudhuij, and Greet Cardon, "Effectiveness and Feasibility of Lowering Playground Density During Recess." *BMC Public Health* 13 (2013): 1154. DOI: 10.1186/1471-2458-13-1154.

33 Anne-Maree Parrish, Don Iverson, Ken Russell, and Heather Yeatman, "Psychosocial Barriers to Playground Activity Levels." *British Journal of School Nursing* 7, no. 3 (2012): 131–7.

34 Yolanda Escalante, Antonio García-Hermoso, Karianne Backx, and Jose M. Saavedra, "Playground Designs to Increase Physical Activity Levels During School Recess: A Systematic Review." *Health Education & Behavior* 41, no. 2 (2014): 138–44.

35 Gareth Stratton and Elaine Mullan, "The Effect of Multicolor Playground Markings on Children's Physical Activity Level During Recess." *Preventive Medicine* 41, no. 5–6 (2005): 828–33.

36 Mine Yildirim, Lauren Arundell, Ester Cerin, Valerie Carson, Helen Brown, David Crawford, Kylie D. Hesketh, Nicola D. Ridgers, Saskia Te Velde, Mai J. M. Chinapaw, and Jo Salmon, "What Helps Children to Move More at School Recess and Lunchtime?" *British Journal of Sports Medicine* 48, no. 3 (2014): 271–7.

37 Karen J. Coleman, Karly S. Geller, Richard R. Rosenkranz, and David A. Dzewaltowski, "Physical Activity and Healthy Eating in the After-School Environment." *Journal of School Health* 78, no. 12 (2008): 633–40.

38 Adam J. Lucas, and Janet E. Dyment, "Where Do Children Choose to Play on the School Ground? The Influence of Green Design." *Education* 3-13 38, no. 2 (2010): 177–89.

39 Kathleen L. Bagot, Felicity Catherine Louise Allen, and Samia Toukhsati, "Perceived Restorativeness of Children's School Playground Environments." *Journal of Environmental Psychology* 41 (2015): 1–9.

40 José A. Corraliza, Silvia Collado, and Lisbeth Bethelmy, "Nature as a Moderator of Stress in Urban Children." *Asia Pacific International Conference on Environment-Behaviour Studies (Aice-Bs)* 38 (2012): 253–63.

41 Fredrika Martensson, Märit Jansson, Maria Johansson, Anders Raustorp, Maria Kylin, and Cecilia Boldemann, "The Role of Greenery for Physical Activity Play at School Grounds." *Urban Forestry & Urban Greening* 13, no. 1 (2014): 103–13.

42 Rebecca J. Sargisson and Ian G. McLean, "Investigating Children's Play Preferences and Safety in New Zealand Playgrounds." *Children, Youth and Environments* 23, no. 2 (2013): 1–21.

43 Karen Martin, Alexandra Bremner, Jo Salmon, Michael Rosenberg, and Billie Giles-Corti, "School and Individual-Level Characteristics Are Associated with Children's Moderate to Vigorous-Intensity Physical Activity during School Recess." *Australian & New Zealand Journal of Public Health* 36, no. 5 (2012): 469–77.

44 Nancy M. Wells, Beth M. Myers, and Charles R. Henderson, "School Gardens and Physical Activity: A Trial of Elementary Schools." *Preventive Medicine* 69, Suppl 1 (2014): S27–33.

45 Leah Frerichs, Jeri Brittin, Dina Sorensen, Matthew J. Trowbridge, Amy L. Yaroch, Mohammad Siapush, Melissa Tibbits, and Terry T. K. Huang, "Influence of School Architecture and Design on Healthy Eating." *American Journal of Public Health* 105, no. 4 (2015): e46–e57.

46 Ramona Robinson-O'Brien, Mary Story, and Stephanie Heim, "Impact of Garden-Based Youth Nutrition Intervention Programs: A Review." *Journal of the American Dietetic Association* 109, no. 2 (2009): 273–80.

47 Dorothy Blair, "The Child in the Garden: An Evaluative Review of the Benefits of School Gardening." *Journal of Environmental Education* 40, no. 2 (2009): 15–38.

48 Zahra Sadat Zomorodian, Mohammad Tahsildoost, and Mohammadreza Hafezi, "Thermal Comfort in Educational Buildings: A Review Article." *Renewable and Sustainable Energy Reviews* 59 (2016): 895–906.

49 Despoina Teli, Patrick A. B. James, and Mark F. Jentsch, "Thermal Comfort in Naturally Ventilated Primary School Classrooms." *Building Research and Information* 41, no. 3 (2013): 301–16.

50 Lia Chatzidiakou, Dejan Mumovic, and Alex Summerfield, "Is CO2 a Good Proxy for Indoor Air Quality in Classrooms?" *Building Services Engineering Research & Technology* 36, no. 2 (2015): 162–81.

51 Mari Turunen, Oluyemi Toyinbo, Tuula Patus, Aino Nevalainen, Richard Shaughnessy, and Ulla Haverinen-Shaughnessy, "Indoor Environmental Quality in School Buildings." *International Journal of Hygiene and Environmental Health* 217, no. 7 (2014): 733–39.

52 Robert Walinder, Kristina Gunnarsson, Roma Runeson, and Greta Smedje, "Physiological and Psychological Stress Reactions in Relation to Classroom Noise." *Scandinavian Journal of Work, Environment & Health* 33, no. 4 (2007): 260–6.

53 Mohammadreza Nilforoushan, Raid Hanna, Hassan Sadeghi Naeini, and Farhang Mozzafar, "Role and Architectural Characteristics in Primary Schools for Day Light in Glasgow (Scotland)." *Review of Higher Education & Self-Learning* 6, no. 20 (2013): 57–66.

54 Valeria De Giuli, Chiara M. Pontarollo, Michele De Carli, and Anotnino Di Bella, "Overall Assessment of Indoor Conditions in a School Building." *International Journal of Environmental Research* 8, no. 1 (2014): 27–38.

55 Mariana Vieira Batistão, Anna Claudia Sentanin, Cristiane Shinohara Moriguchi, Gert-ÅkeHansson, Helenice Jane Cote Gil Coury, and Tatiana de Oliveira Sato, "Furniture Dimensions and Postural Overload for Schoolchildren" *Work* 41 (2012): 4817–24.

56 Georgia Panagiotopoulou, Kosmas Christoulas, Anthoula Papanckolaou, and Konstantinos Mandroukas, "Classroom Furniture Dimensions and Anthropometric Measures in Primary School." *Applied ergonomics* 35, no. 2 (2004): 121–28.

57 Pedro Ferreira Reis, Antonio Renato Pereira Moro, J. Placido Da Silva, Luis Paschoarelli, Francisco Nunes Sobrinho, and L. Peres "Anthropometric Aspects of Body Seated in School." *Work* 41 (2012): 907–14.

58 C. S. Savanur, C.R. Altekar, and Amitabha De, "Lack of Conformity Between Indian Classroom Furniture and Student Dimensions." *Ergonomics* 50, no. 10 (2007): 1612–25.

59 Mohamed Zaki Ramadan, "Does Saudi School Furniture Meet Ergonomics Requirements?" *Work* 38, no. 2 (2011): 93–101.

60 Maria Antonia Gonçalves, and Pedro M. Arezes, "Postural Assessment of School Children." *Work* 41 (2012): 876–80.

61 Greet Cardon, Dirk De Clercq, Ilse De Bourdeaudhuij, and Dieter Breithecker, "Sitting Habits in Elementary Schoolchildren." *Patient Education and Counseling* 54, no. 2 (2004): 133–42.

62 Saeideh Aminian, Erica A. Hinckson, and Tom Stewart, "Modifying the Classroom Environment to Increase Standing and Reduce Sitting." *Building Research & Information* 43, no. 5 (2015): 631–45.

63 Mark E. Benden, Jamilia J. Blake, Monica L. Wendel, and John C. Huber, "The Impact of Stand-Biased Desks in Classrooms on Calorie Expenditure in Children." *American Journal of Public Health* 101, no. 8 (2011): 1433–36.

64 Mark E. Benden, Hongwei Zhao, Christina E. Jeffrey, Monica L. Wendel, and Jamilia J. Blake, "The Evaluation of the Impact of a Stand-Biased Desk on Energy Expenditure and Physical Activity for Elementary School Students." *International Journal of Environmental Research and Public Health* 11, no. 9 (2014): 9361–75.

65 Jamilia J. Blake, Mark E. Benden, and Monica L. Wendel, "Using Stand/Sit Workstations in Classrooms." *Journal of Public Health Management and Practice* 18, no. 5 (2012): 412–15.

66 Erica A. Hinckson, Saeideh Aminian, Erica Ikeda, Tom Stewart, Melody Oliver, Scott Duncan, and Grant Schofield, "Acceptability of Standing Workstations in Elementary Schools." *Preventive Medicine* 56, no. 1 (2013): 82–85.

67 Lorraine Lanningham-Foster, Randal C. Foster, Shelly K. McCrady, Chinmay U. Manohar, Teresa B. Jensen, Naim G. Mitre, James O. Hill, and James A. Levine, "Changing the School Environment to Increase Physical Activity in Children." *Obesity* 16, no. 8 (2008): 1849–53.

68 Andrew James Williams, Katrina Mary Wyatt, Alison Jane Hurts, and Craig Anthony Williams, "A Review of Associations between the Primary School Built Environment and Childhood Overweight and Obesity." *Health & Place* 18, no. 3 (2012): 504–14.

69 Marcella Ucci, Stephen Law, Richard Andrews, Abi Fisher, Lee Smith, Alexia Sawyer, and Alexi Marmot, "Indoor School Environments, Physical Activity, Sitting Behaviour and Pedagogy: A Scoping Review." *Building Research & Information* 43, no. 5 (2015): 566–81.

70 By Stu Ryan and Lisa Lucks Mendel, "Acoustics in Physical Education Settings." *Educational Facility Planner* 44, no. 4 (2010): 38–43.

71 Meenakshi Fernandes and Roland Sturm, "Facility Provision in Elementary Schools." *Preventive Medicine* 50 (2010): S30–S35.

72 Jennifer L. Huberty, Danae Dinkel, Jason Coleman, Aaron Beighle, and Bettye Apenteng, "The Role of Schools in Children's Physical Activity Participation: Staff Perceptions." *Health Education Research* 27, no. 6 (2012): 986–95.

73 Alessandro Rigolon, and Maxine Alloway, "Children and Their Development as the Starting Point: A New Way to Think About the Design of Elementary Schools." *Educational and Child Psychology* 28, no. 1 (2011): 64–76.

74 Shelly K. McCrady-Spitzer, Chinmay U. Manohar, Gabriel A. Koepp, and James A. Levine, "Low-Cost and Scalable Classroom Equipment to Promote Physical Activity and Improve Education." *Journal Physical Activity and Health* 12, no. 9 (2014): 1259–63. DOI: 101.123/jpah.2014–0159.

75 Katherine Bathgate and Andrea Begley, "What Perth Parents Think About Food for School Lunch Boxes." *Nutrition & Dietetics* 68, no. 1 (2011): 21–6.

76 Ethan A. Bergman, Nancy S. Buergel, Timothy F. Englund, and Annaka Femrite, "The Relationship Between the Length of the Lunch Period and Nutrient Consumption in the Elementary School Lunch Setting." *The Journal of Child Nutrition & Management* 28, no. 2 (2004) http://docs.schoolnutrition.org/newsroom/jcnm/04fall/bergman/bergman2.asp.

77 Sue N. Moore, Simon Murphy, Katy Tapper, and Laurence Moore, "The Social, Physical and Temporal Characteristics of Primary School Dining Halls and Their Implications for Children's Eating Behaviours." *Health Education* 110, no. 5 (2010): 399–411.

78 Rachana Bhatt, "Timing Is Everything: The Impact of School Lunch Length on Children's Body Weight." *Southern Economic Journal* 80, no. 3 (2014): 656–76.

79 Wendelin M. Slusser, William G. Cumberland, Ben L. Browdy, Linda Lange, and Charlotte Neumann, "A School Salad Bar Increases Frequency of Fruit and Vegetable Consumption among Children." *Public Health Nutrition* 10, no. 12 (2007): 1490–96.

80 Rebecca Muckelbauer, Kerstin Clausen, and Mathilde Kersting, "Long-Term Process Evaluation of a School-Based Program for Overweight Prevention." *Child Care Health and Development* 35, no. 6 (2009): 851–7.

81 Terry T-K. Huang, Dina Sorensen, Steven Davis, Leah Frerichs, Jerri Brittin, Joseph Celentano, Kelly Callahan, and Matthew Trowbridge, "Peer Reviewed: Healthy Eating

Design Guidelines for School Architecture." *Preventing Chronic Disease* 10 (2013). DOI: http://dx.doi.org/10.5888/pcd10.120084.

82 See namely the books: Peter C. Lippman, *Evidenced-Based Design of Elementary and Secondary Schools*. New York: Wiley, 2010; Bradford Perkins and Raymond Bordwell, *Building Type Basics for Elementary, Secondary Schools*. New York: Wiley, 2002, 2nd ed. 2009 or OWP/P Architects + VS Furniture + Brice Mau Design. *The Third Teacher*. New York: Abrams, 2010. A few books were also written to inform school architectural programming. See C. Kenneth Tanner and Jeff A. Lackney, *Educational Facilities Planning: Leadership, Architecture, and Management*. New York: Allyn & Bacon, 2006. Some books address the future of educational facilities. See Rotraut Walden, *Schools for the Future: Design Proposals From Architectural Psychology*. Berlin: Springer, 2015; Nair Prakash, *Blueprint for Tomorrow: Redesigning Schools for Student-Centered Learning*. Cambridge, MA: Harvard Education PR, 2014, or Peter Barrett et al. *Clever Classroom*. Summary report of the Head Project, Manchester, School of the Built Environment. Manchester: University of Salford, 2015. Finally, some relevant chapters targeting schools: see Dak Kopec, "Learning and Education." In *Environmental Psychology for Design*, 213–34. Singapore: Fairchild, 2006, 2nd ed. 2010; or Sandra Horne Martin, "The Classroom Environment and the Children's Performance." In *Children and Their Environments: Learning, Using and Designing Spaces*, edited by C. Spencer and M. Blades, 91–108. Cambridge: Cambridge University Press, 2006.

83 For examples of strategies developed at the School of Architecture of Laval University in Canada to integrate people-environment research to the teaching of undergraduate and graduate design studios, see Carole Després and Denise Piché, "Linking People Environment and Design: What Is Missing?" In *Handbook of Environmental Psychology and Quality of Life Research*, edited by Ghozlane Fleury-Bahi, Enric Pol, and Oscar Navarro, 65–84. Berlin: Springer, 2016.

11

UNIVERSAL DESIGN, DESIGN FOR AGING IN PLACE, AND HABILITATIVE DESIGN IN RESIDENTIAL ENVIRONMENTS

Jon A. Sanford and Shauna Corry Hernandez

Introduction

Today, consumers of all ages and abilities want to live, work and play in healthy, supportive environments that are well designed, function for their needs and abilities and enhance well-being. In residential applications, designers and manufacturers seek to address the functional limitations of older adults and people with disabilities through a variety of design philosophies including Universal Design practices, Aging in Place initiatives and Habilitative Design. While each philosophy meets a different level of specificity of user needs, thoughtful application of a design strategy based on specific situational needs can result in highly supportive and often long-term living environments. Determining how effective each philosophy could be for a user is an important consideration for the designer, one that could either positively or negatively impact the user for the rest of his or her life.

Although all three design strategies are intended to meet users' needs, the approaches are hierarchical, from addressing the accessibility and usability needs of many to individual residents themselves. Of the three strategies, Universal Design represents the most global approach to meeting usability needs. It is an all-encompassing and inclusive design strategy that focuses on design for all users, to the greatest extent possible.[1] As such, universal design intends to meet the needs of people with functional limitations, including older adults and people with disabilities, through the design of everyday products, devices and spaces that would be used by the general population of people without limitations. Clearly, this scattershot approach to designing environments that are as inclusive as possible is not intended to address either the individual functional needs of specific dwelling occupants or the common needs of a particular user group, such as older adults, that are shared by those occupants.

To address the typical functional limitations that are shared by older adults as a group, such as poor gait, balance, strength, stamina, hearing and sight, Aging in

Place is a design strategy that has been shown to be highly effective in addressing the specific needs that are associated with those limitations, including grab bars and hand rails for support, ramps and lifts to eliminate stair climbing and increased light to facilitate seeing. Despite the more tailored approach for an older adult population, aging in place is still based on generally accepted understanding of functional needs of a broad user group. It is not individualized to the specific situational needs of an individual occupant or occupants of a residential environment. Like universal design, aging in place may not adequately address an individual user or users' situational needs.

Habilitative Design, on the other hand, is a philosophy that focuses on design to meet occupants' specific functional and situational needs. As a result, this approach will produce a highly individualized and customized residential environment. The process of determining what elements of each philosophy to use as guiding principles when promoting health and well-being through design in residential environments is the focus of this chapter.

The Origins of Residential Design to Meet Functional Needs

History of Accessible Design

Few design theories and practices recognize diversity of human form and function.[2] To the extent that typical everyday designs of buildings, spaces and objects are based on human ability at all, they are based on technical standards and dimensions of "normal" body structure, function and capacities.[3] For people with disabilities, who tend to have less than "normal" abilities, everyday design exerts demands that often exceed their abilities. The result is design barriers to accessibility and usability.

To remove or overcome design barriers for people with functional limitations, specialized accessible designs have traditionally been added to everyday designs. Acting as enablers or facilitators that address barriers created by everyday designs, specialized designs serve as prosthetic supports to improve function compensating for specific limitations in ability. For example, a ramp compensates for an inability to ambulate or lift one's leg whereas grab bars compensate for loss of ability to raise and lower oneself. With the assistance of specialized designs, everyday design that is disabling can become enabling, allowing many individuals with disabilities to carry out basic activities associated with daily living safely and independently.

The origins of specialized accessible design in the U.S. can be traced to the period following World War II and continuing through the ensuing wars in Korea and Vietnam. During this period, there was a dramatic growth in the population of people with disabilities driven by the return of veterans with war-related injuries. The mismatch between the needs and abilities of large numbers of impaired war veterans highlighted the need to build accessible environments that would enable these individuals to work, attend school and live an active life. The result was the development of accessibility standards and guidelines accompanied by a series of legislative acts beginning in the early 1960s.[4] This included the first (1961) version of the American National Standards Institute (ANSI) *A 117.1—Making Buildings Accessible to and Usable by the Physically Handicapped*, a consensus standard which is now promulgated by the International Code Council. ANSI A117.1 was followed by the U.S. Architectural Barriers Act of 1968, which, among other things, established the U.S. Architectural and Transportation Barriers Accessibility Board (now known as the Access Board) to develop the Minimum Guidelines and Requirements for Accessible Design (MGRAD) to ensure that federally-funded buildings and transportation options were accessible to people with disabilities.[5]

The 1970s and 1980s brought further transformational legislation to improve accessibility for people with disabilities including amendments to the Architectural Barriers Act in 1970 and 1976, Section 504 of the Rehabilitation Act of 1973, the Individuals with Disabilities Education Act of 1975 and the Fair Housing Amendments Act of 1988. Although the needs of veterans resulted in legislation to provide accessible facilities in federal buildings and those of organizations that received federal funding, it took the Disabilities Rights movement almost another quarter century to push through legislation that would guarantee equal rights for people with disabilities, including equal access to public facilities, transportation, education and the workplace.

These efforts culminated in the passage of the historic Americans with Disabilities Act (ADA) in 1990, which was the first piece of national legislation in any country to insure equal rights for people with disabilities. Among the various pieces of the Act, Title III mandated the Access Board to develop accessibility guidelines for all public facilities. First published in 1991, the ADA Accessibility Guidelines for Public Accommodations and Commercial Facilities were originally based on the MGRAD. With new amendments to the ADA in 2010, a major revision was made to Title III to reconcile the new ADA Amendments Act Standards with ANSI A177.1.[6]

Defining the parameters of the ADA:

> The ADA is one of America's most comprehensive pieces of civil rights legislation that prohibits discrimination and guarantees that people with disabilities have the same opportunities as everyone else to participate in the mainstream of American life—to enjoy employment opportunities, to purchase goods and services, and to participate in State and local government programs and services. Modeled after the Civil Rights Act of 1964, which prohibits discrimination on the basis of race, color, religion, sex, or national origin—and Section 504 of the Rehabilitation Act of 1973—the ADA is an "equal opportunity" law for people with disabilities.
>
> *(U.S. Department of Justice Civil Rights Division 2015)*[7]

Because of the significance of the ADA and its associated accessibility guidelines, it is not surprising that most definitions of accessible design,[8,9] including accessible housing, link accessibility to compliance with requirements associated with the

ADA, even though the guidelines only apply to public facilities. Nonetheless, while housing accessibility is not mandated to comply with ADA accessibility standards, specifications within the Standards, such as types and sizes of grab bars and slopes of ramps, are typically used as the basis for accessible design in home environments.

The Disillusion of Accessible Design

Intentionally, accessible design is a prosthetic, specialized design that compensates for deficiencies in everyday design through a reduction or elimination of usability barriers for individuals with limitations in specific types of abilities. For example, to cross a street, curb ramps assist individuals in wheelchairs, whereas auditory crosswalk signals help people who are blind. Accessible design is, by nature, a reactive approach that is added on to everyday products and building features. As Band-Aids, specialized designs are often institutional-looking and stand out. Thus, although they enable everyday design, they are often associated with the stigma of disability and institutional care.[10]

For individuals with functional limitations who are already predisposed to being stigmatized because their abilities are different than the general population, specialized designs, many of which were originally designed for institutional settings (e.g., hospitals) and are medical in appearance, reinforce societal stereotypes by emphasizing and directing attention to these differences in public or residential settings. As a result, accessible design is equally an object of stigma as the traits from which the stigma is derived.

Universal Design

The need for less stigmatizing accommodations and more aesthetically pleasing and functional products designed for all users, not just people with disabilities, led Ron Mace, an architect as well as an individual with a disability and a staunch advocate of accessible design, to promulgate the concept of universal design.[11–13] Although the concept first began to emerge in the late 1980s, Mace's ideas were fittingly first published in 1991, the same year as the initial ADA Accessibility Guidelines. The definition of universal design included in that first publication is still the most generally accepted definition of universal design today. In that seminal work, Mace defined universal design as: "the design of products and environments to be useable by all people, to the greatest extent possible, without the need for adaptation or specialized design."[14]

Conceptually, universal design does not view disability as a single point requiring specialized intervention, but a continuum of ability that would benefit from more supportive everyday design. It is an approach to design that accommodates the widest possible range of body shapes, dimensions and movements through contextually appropriate mainstream design solutions.[15] Moreover, by making everyday designs more useable for as many people as possible, universal design not only has built-in accessibility, but accessibility is undetectable.[16]

The Case for Universal Design

In the half century that has passed since the development of the early accessibility guidelines, the demographics of the population as a whole has changed dramatically. By most criteria, over 10 percent of the U.S. population has some limitation in ability. Using the broadest category of functional limitations of any kind as a basis, (e.g., traveling three city blocks or hearing typical conversation), more than 50 percent of the U.S. population could be characterized as having diminished abilities.[17]

Although older people are living longer and in better health, they typically have limitations in one or more functional abilities. Similarly, a larger number of individuals are living longer with increasingly diverse and complex types of disabilities. Not surprisingly, a considerable amount of research over the past three decades has shown that accessible design does not adequately compensate for the range of functional limitations and comorbidities that are common among older adults, including limitations in strength, stamina, reach, lifting legs and sit-to-stand or the types of secondary conditions that are common among people aging with disabilities. In fact, there is a direct relationship between age and functional limitation. While the rate of activity limitation is around 40 percent for the population 65 years or over, it increases to almost 60 percent for those 85 or over.

More generally, everyone experiences some type(s) of activity limitation(s) during their lifetime. These can be intrinsic due to body stature, such as being short or tall, which impact reaching things up high or low, respectively. They can be temporary due to a health condition, pregnancy or injury, such as a broken leg that limits mobility, causes fatigue or reduces stamina and they can change from day to day due to variations in ability, such as poor processing ability caused by a lack of sleep. They can also be caused by extrinsic situational factors such as unfamiliarity with the way an appliance operates, which prevents its use, a parent pushing a stroller that can't go up or down steps or someone carrying a package that prevents use of one's arms. Finally, temporary disability can be caused by extrinsic environmental factors, such as a dark room that limits sight or excessive noise that limits hearing.

Unlike accessible design, which addresses different types of functional limitations independent of each other, thus creating a variety of specialized products and environmental features, universal design considers the range of human abilities/limitations at one time in the design of everyday products and environments. As a result, a universal design approach is useful in residential environments, not only in supporting individuals and their families across their lifespan, but also in supporting different people and their families across the lifespan of the home. Most importantly, universal design is everyday design. By accommodating users' functional needs into everyday design, accessibility and usability are invisible, thus avoiding the stigma of specialized design. In the end, users, both with disabilities and those without, interior designers, architects, builders and building managers all want products and accommodations that make life easier and richer for everyone.[18]

Design for Aging in Place

Despite the obvious benefits of universal design, it is not a panacea. While it represents a holistic approach to the design of housing that is supportive of the range of human functional needs, it cannot realistically address all needs of all people all the time. It can set a baseline for usability that will reduce, to the greatest extent possible, the need for more customized designs that are more tailored to individual functional needs. For older adults, who share common age-related functional limitations, design for aging in place—the practice of modifying one's existing home to address changing needs unique to older adults—is a strategy that provides a first pass at that customization.

History of Aging in Place

Over the past 50 years, the aging tsunami has hit the U.S. and much of the industrialized world, swelling the number of people 65+ living at home in the community. According to the U.S. Census Bureau, by 2020 there will be almost 54 million people over 65 years of age, an increase of more than 50 million from the 1900 Census. Much of the growth can be attributed to the aging of the Baby Boom generation. The first wave of boomers (born 1946–1954), who turned 65 years old five years ago, have now just passed age 70. The second wave of late boomers or trailing edge boomers born between 1955 and 1965 will begin turning 65 in 2020.[19]

Although the needs of older adults have been a concern for hundreds of years,[20] the concept of aging in place is at the forefront today not only because of the large number of people it affects,[21] but also because the way society embraces aging has changed. Whereas family, religious groups and fraternal organizations often met the needs of prior generations while they remained in the community, older adults were often moved to institutional facilities when those needs could no longer be met. It was only with the Older Americans Act (OAA) of 1965 that rights for suitable housing and independence in managing life pursuits were addressed, along with issues including adequate income and access to health care.[22]

It is the housing needs of baby boomers and trailing edge boomers that frame the discussion of aging in place. Boomers regard institutionalization, represented by traditional skilled nursing homes to which many saw their grandparents relocated, as particularly loathsome. Not surprisingly, 89 percent of boomers wish to remain in their homes and choose to remain living independently.[23,24,25]

Unfortunately, many homes are not designed to provide support to meet the needs of older adults. Physical barriers in the home are common and pervasive[26] and are the primary source of misfit between the needs of community-dwelling seniors and the places in which they live. Barriers, such as stairs, narrow doorways, poor lighting, lack of visual contrast, shower curbs or tub sidewalls, low toilets, narrow halls and doors, small spaces and inefficient layout can create physical hazards and social isolation that can put community-dwelling individuals with functional limitations at significant risk for adverse health events, such as falls and injuries, difficulty in performing ADLs (Activities of Daily Living), loss of independence, depression, inactivity and obesity.[27,28] The design of homes of older adults can also make it difficult to accommodate their health care needs, including types of health care equipment and their care providers.

Aging in place is a design strategy that enables older Americans to stay in their own communities, among friends and strong support networks[29,30] by modifying homes to address the changing needs of the occupants as they age. Like accessible design, design for aging in place includes specific modifications that are tailored to the functional needs of the population. However, unlike accessible design, which is based on the same design for individuals with the same singular need (e.g., a ramp for wheelchair users), modifications for aging in place consider many different designs for individuals who have many simultaneous needs, such as the addition of toilet grab bars and a contrasting color for the seat for someone who has both a loss of strength and balance, but also a loss of contrast sensitivity.[31]

Benefits of Aging in Place

Living independently in a familiar environment allows aging adults freedom, increased comfort and safety, and can seriously impact their financial situation. Maintaining independence, specifically in the context of design, contributes to a safe and supportive living environment and increases the likelihood of an aging adult remaining in their home.[32,33,34]

Remaining at home also has strong financial benefits for aging adults.[35] With the high cost of other living options including assisted care facilities, the ability to stay at home not only saves money, but is considered to be good for mental and emotional health. HUD notes that many aging Americans are choosing to remain in place because it is an affordable option. For seniors who own their own home, or participate in home equity conversion mortgages, the cost of remaining in place is often feasible even with in-home care when compared to living in an assisted care facility. The cost of living in an assisted care facility is three times more than non-institutional or at home care, and for over 94 percent of seniors the cost is paid for out of pocket.[36] One study conducted in the U.S.[37] comparing Medicare and Medicaid programs for seniors using an aging in place long-term care program consisting of home and community-based health care services to those living in a nursing home found that the former group had potential savings of $1,591.61 per month.

Habilitative Design

Homes vary widely in their location, size, condition and physical design characteristics. Similarly, the needs of people with a variety of functional limitations vary widely. The success of housing as a supportive, needs-meeting setting is, therefore, more complicated than simply adding a ramp to the front of house or grab bars around the toilet. It involves a diverse set of contextual factors (i.e., physical, social, cultural and policy environments and personal factors) as well as an array of individualized rehabilitation interventions that go beyond baseline usability needs of universal design and the generic population needs of older adults addressed by aging in place, especially those users with a cognitive disability.[38]

Habilitative design is a relatively new design philosophy that provides more individualized design by focusing on the unique daily living needs of individuals that will enable them to function at their highest capacity. Because of the idiosyncratic nature of an individual's needs, the outcome of habilitative design is a customized environment.

The concept of habilitative design comes from the health care world of disability and rehabilitation where the goal of most therapies is to either keep or regain independence. Rehabilitation health care services focus on helping an individual regain a mental or physical skill or ability lost through an accident or illness. Habilitation health care services focus on teaching patients new skills or abilities. Habilitation therapy was first applied in 1996 by dementia researchers Joanne Koenig-Coste and Paul Raia, who sought to enhance life quality for patients with Alzheimer's disease by focusing on what the patient could do at any given time during the illness, rather than on what the patient couldn't do.[39] The goal of all habilitation therapies is to help occupants gain maximum skill levels and abilities within their living environments. Habilitative design is used at a basic level by Occupational Therapists as part of the environmental modification process and is often unique to every client or group household. According to Kopec,[40] architects and interior designers are better suited to address habilitative design needs because designers have environmental modification skills that go beyond basic needs and decoration.

The principles of habilitative design include the maintenance of personal safety while maximizing independence and basic freedoms, accommodation of an individual's unique abilities, addressing unique challenges in the environment, retaining a residential atmosphere despite the need for medical equipment and the use of materials and fixtures that withstand or minimize negative outcomes from behavioral actions. Habilitative design has three cardinal rules.[41]

1. Each occupant should have complete and unencumbered access to all areas within their homes.
2. Designs should blend into the environment and should never call attention, or lead a casual visitor to know that a person with differing or limited abilities resides in that home.
3. Predictive modeling should be used to enhance health and safety through the anticipation of probable unintended outcomes.

In contrast to universal design, habilitative design is typically applied to a residential design for a specific individual or a group of occupants with specific sets of limitations, often including cognitive in nature. Also, unlike design for aging in place, habilitative design does not come complete with a preset kit of parts (e.g., ramps, grab bars and tub transfer benches). Rather, habilitative design strives for unique design solutions that are situationally-driven by the needs of the users and the demands of the context. Thus, whereas universal design is highly replicable for all users, and the design for aging in place is highly replicable for the target population, these strategies may not reliably address all user needs. In contrast, because habilitative design addresses unique situational needs, design solutions are not replicable, but very reliant on the needs of each identified user.

Conclusion

Designers are uniquely qualified to lead the assessment and application of design strategies that address universal needs, needs related to aging and the needs of specific people with specific conditions. What makes the design professional uniquely suited to the lead these design initiatives are the designer's understanding of space and human perceptions of that space, color perception and cognition and how color can effect neural stimulation, optical illusions and faulty depth perception.[42]

Whether one is designing several retail stores that will be replicated through many diverse geographies, designing local or national retirement communities or developing congregate or residential housing for specific populations there are three common threads: designs that support people, designs that are based on sets of situations or conditions and enhancing quality of life for all. To this end, design and design practitioners are moving toward greater operationalization of health and well-being, through an integrated approach to human physical, psychological and sociological health as they relate with the human occupation of our built environments. This thus affords the designer an unprecedented ability to be included as a vital part of the clinical, social and environmental health care team.

Notes

1 Ron Mace, Grame Hardie, and Jaine Place, "Accessible Environments: Toward Universal Design," in *Innovation by Design*, ed. Edward T. White (New York: Van Nostrand Reinhold Publishers, 1991), 155–175.
2 Rob Imrie, "From Universal to Inclusive Design in the Built Environment," in *Disabling Barriers—Enabling Environments*, eds. John Swain, Sally French, Colin Barnes, and Charles C. Thomas (London: Sage Publications, 2004), 279–284.
3 Ibid.
4 Polly Welch and Chris Palames, "A Brief History of Disability Rights Legislation in the United States," in *Strategies for Teaching Universal Design*, ed. Polly Welch (Boston, MA: Adaptive Environments Center, 1995), 5–12.
5 Ibid.
6 "ADA Standards for Accessible Design," Information and Technical Assistance on the Americans With Disability Act, United States Department of Justice and Civil Rights Division, www.ada.gov/2010ADAstandards_index.htm.
7 "Introduction to the ADA," Information and Technical Assistance on the Americans With Disability Act, United States Department of Justice and Civil Rights Division, www.ada.gov/ada_intro.htm.
8 Robert F. Erlandson, *Universal and Accessible Design of Products, Services and Processes* (Boca Raton: CRC Press, 2008).

9   John P. S. Salmen, "U.S. Accessibility Codes and Standards: Challenges for Universal Design," in *Universal Design Handbook*, eds. Wolfgang F. E. Preiser and Elaine Ostroff (New York: McGraw-Hill, 2001), 12.1–12.8.

10 Jon A. Sanford, *Design for the Ages: Universal Design as a Rehabilitation Strategy* (New York: Springer, 2012).

11 Cynthia Leibrock and Susan Behar, *Beautiful Barrier-Free: A Visual Guide to Accessibility* (Hoboken: Wiley, 1992).

12 Polly Welch, *Strategies for Teaching Universal Design* (Boston, MA: Adaptive Environments Center, 1995).

13 Wolfgang F. E. Preiser and Elaine Ostroff, *Universal Design Handbook* (New York: McGraw-Hill, 2001).

14 Ron Mace, Grame Hardie, and Jaine Place, "Accessible Environments.".

15 Imrie, "From Universal to Inclusive Design.".

16 Sanford, *Design for the Ages*.

17 Gary S. Danford and Beth Tauke, *Universal Design New York* (New York: New York City Mayor's Office for People with Disabilities, 2001).

18 Shauna Corry Hernandez, "Exploring the Schism: Toward an Empathetic Language," in *The Handbook of Interior Design*, eds. JoAnn Asher Thompson and Nancy Blossom (Malden: Wiley, 2015), 148–170.

19 "Aging in the United States: Past Present and Future," U.S. Department of Commerce, Economics and Statistics Administration, Bureau of the Census, www.census.gov/population/international/files/97agewc.pdf.

20 W. Andrew Achenbaum and L. Christian Carr, "A Brief History of Aging Services in the United States," *Generations, Journal of the American Society of Aging* (July 7, 2014), www.asaging.org/blog/brief-history-aging-services-united-states.

21 Daniel DiClerico, "10 Questions... Michael Thomas, Aging in Place Expert," *Consumer Reports News*, November 4, 2008, www.consumerreports.org/cro/news/2008/11/10-questions-for-michael-thomas-aging-in-place-expert/index.htm.

22 Achenbaum and Carr, "A Brief History of Aging Services.".

23 Dak Kopec, *Health, Sustainability, and the Built Environment* (New York: Fairchild, 2008).

24 Achenbaum and Carr, *A Brief History of Aging Services*.

25 "Aging in Place: Facilitating Choice and Independence," Evidence Matters, U.S. Department of Housing and Urban Development, 2013, www.huduser.gov/portal/periodicals/em/fall13/highlight2.html.

26 Thomas M. Gill, Christianna S. Williams, J.T. Robinson, and Mary E. Tinetti, "Mismatches Between the Home Environment and Physical Capabilities Among Community-Living Older Persons," *Journal of the American Geriatrics Society* 47 (1999): 88–92.

27 "Falls Among Older Adults: An Overview," Centers for Disease Control and Prevention, May 30, 2012, www.cdc.gov/HomeandRecreationalSafety/Falls/adultfalls.html.

28 Julianne Holt-Lunstad, Timothy B. Smith, and J. Bradley Layton, "Social Relationships and Mortality Risk: A Meta-Analytic Review," *PLoS Medicine* 7, no. 7 (2010): e1000316, doi:10.1371/journal.pmed.1000316.

29 Drue Lawlor and Michael A. Thomas, *Residential Design for Aging in Place* (Hoboken: Wiley, 2008).

30 Esther Iecovich, "Aging in Place: From Theory to Practice," *Anthropological Notebooks* 20, no. 1 (2014): 21–33.

31 Kopec, *Health, Sustainability*.

32 DiClerico, "10 Questions."

33 Lawlor and Thomas, *Residential Design for Aging*.

34 Iecovich, "Aging in Place."

35 "Measuring the Costs and Savings of Aging in Place," Evidence Matters, U.S. Department of Housing and Urban Development, 2013, www.huduser.gov/portal/periodicals/em/fall13/highlight2.html.

36 HUD, "Measuring the Costs."

37 Karen Marek, Frank Stetzer, Scott Adams, Lori Popejoy, and Marilyn Rantz, "Aging in Place Versus Nursing Home Care: Comparison of Costs to Medicare and Medicaid," *Research*

in Gerontological Nursing 5, no. 2 (2012): 123–129, doi:10.3928/19404921-20110802-01, https://eldertech.missouri.edu/files/Papers/Rantz/The%20continued%20success%20of%20registered%20nurse%20care%20coordination.pdf.

38 Dak Kopec, "How a Team of Students Transformed a Group Home Into a Haven Through Habilitative Design," *Inhabitat*, May 8, 2015, http://inhabitat.com/tag/habilitative-design/.

39 Paul Raia, "Habilitation Therapy: A New Starscape," in *Enhancing the Quality of Life in Advanced Dementia*, eds. Ladislav Volicer and Lisa Bloom-Charette (Philadelphia, PA: Brunner/Mazel, 2013), 21–34.

40 Kopec, "Habilitative Design."

41 Ibid.

42 Ibid.

12

EMPATHIC DESIGN MATTERS

Moira Gannon Denson

Introduction

Empathic design is a methodology (without a widely established definition) traditionally applied to creating better products, services, and technologies. Though not a mainstream term in the fields of interior design and architecture, those employing empathic design seek a deeper understanding of the users' perspective by targeting the customer's emotions and experiences. In so doing, they improve the health within the spaces they create or design.

Strategies for employing empathic design generally fit into three categories:

- techniques to become immersed in the user's perspective;
- techniques to step back from the user's world to gain a new perspective, giving the user room to own the project; and
- techniques to systematically balance subjective and objective strategies to fulfill increasingly complex project requirements.

Sim Van der Ryn, architect, educator, and researcher, in *Design for an Empathic World: Reconnecting People, Nature, and Self*,[1] cautiously suggests that empathic design is not a standard architectural practice. Empathy requires human-centered design that takes into account the end user's needs including emotional and physical health, and how one links to others and to nature.

Human-centered design (HCD) begins with the users it serves and includes them in the planning for the spaces they will inhabit. Van der Ryn sees this as the starting point for an empathic approach. Aligning empathic design within the broader field of HCD suggests a core emphasis on human needs. Mullaney et al. further expand on human-centered design, sometimes also called user-centered design (UCD), or people-centered design.[2] Their approach shows how design can meet individuals' needs. This chapter explores techniques employed in empathic design that differentiate it from HCD or UCD. Although related to many practices within design, the "way" that they are applied suggests an empathic-design approach.

Empathic design stems from the early developments of *Einfuhlung* (translated as "empathy") by the late nineteenth-century German aesthetic philosophers. Howe explains that by using empathy to feel our way into an artwork, we increase our understanding and appreciation of it.[3] These early philosophers suggested that an empathic experience with art, both as an artist and a viewer, deepens how we look at life and has potential therapeutic value. Design techniques that early on "feel into" the users' experiences can bring innovative-design solutions to spaces, which help to improve users' health and well-being.

Contemporary cultural thinker, Roman Krznaric, in *Empathy: Why It Matters, and How to Get It*, explains that the current explosion of interest in empathy is due to scientific discoveries about human nature.[4] He highlights recent research in child psychology—that three-year-olds demonstrate the ability to see another's perspective by stepping outside themselves. He also cites studies of animals becoming cooperative and empathic as they evolved. Discoveries in neuroscience show our brains consist of a complex empathic circuit, which, if damaged, can affect our empathy toward another. These findings emphasize the need for empathy and of understanding and relating to others as a central concept within our current thinking. Therefore, they should play a significant role in how design responds to societal needs.

Although sometimes mistakenly categorized together, empathy differs from sympathy. According to Kouprie and Visser, sympathy is our concern about the other person's well-being as though you were the other.[5] By contrast, empathy means understanding the other person. According to Howe, sympathy can result in identifying as the user or even projecting onto the user.[6] This does not keep the user's best interest at the front. Therefore, sympathy is problematic for design. Understanding, rather than relating to the user, is more important in the design process.

Immersion

Leonard and Rayport built the concept of empathic design for NPD in the 1990s through techniques that see empathic design as observation in the user's native environment or everyday life.[7] Using field observations, one can gather, analyze, and apply information found in the field. This type of research is very different from traditional NPD-user research because it is not conducted in isolation from other disciplines. Rather, it requires interdisciplinary collaboration.

One such observation method involves shadowing to understand the user's experience. Along with detailed observation and documentation, the shadowing observer also may directly question the user to gain further insight. Observation as an empathic-design strategy allows designers to become informed. It is a good starting point for stepping into the user's world. However, to understand the user's world fully, designers must truly immerse themselves in the user's experience, and may need to take personal risks.

Thomas and McDonagh identify the importance of immersive experiences to expand our understanding and knowledge, outside of our own comfort zones.[8] The technique of *empathic modeling* helps designers use deep insight beyond comfort boundaries to solve problems based on the user's perceived needs. By understanding their own body, designers can understand how others relate to the physical world. This would allow the designer to gain empathy and have an emotional connection with another person.

One of the most well-known demonstrations of empathic modeling is the immersive experience of Patricia Moore, a junior designer in the office of renowned industrial designer Raymond Loewy. Ms. Moore spent 1979–1982 engaged in deep empathic strategies. According to Coleman, Lebbin, and Myerson, Moore went across the U.S. and Canada, visiting more than 100 areas disguised as a woman in her eighties.[9] She altered her body with prosthetics and through empathic modeling created a research base for much inclusive design and universal design practice. She realized that the world was not just divided into the able-bodied and disabled. Rather, we are all 'differently abled.' Throughout our lifetimes, our capabilities change. Moore's social experiment to live as someone much older than herself helped to bring attention to immersive research as a way for product designers to better understand the users.

Interior design and architecture also provide examples of the empathic strategy of immersing oneself in another's daily living to better understand the users' experience. Marika Shioiri-Clark, one of the founders of Boston-based MASS (Model of Architecture Serving Society) Design Group publicly defined what *empathic architecture* meant to her practice of architecture.[10] Designers embedded themselves in the community. They lived onsite. They got to know the client because they became the client. Full immersion and becoming the client may sound complicated, and it certainly means a commitment. MASS Design Group formed their practice as the result of their first major project, the Butaro Hospital in Rwanda. The designers moved to Rwanda, lived onsite, and became a part of the community fabric, ultimately reaching better design outcomes through their immersive methods.

The designer faces many challenges to full participation or use of immersion strategies. The extensive time commitment given to the process of MASS Design Group and Moore's study is generally not possible for most design-research schedules. Often, the client may not want to pay for the designer's research time. Clients may perceive the process as risky and challenging to privacy regulations. Others question whether immersion is truly possible for an architect or designer. Kolko suggests true empathy is unachievable because you are not that person and cannot feel what someone else feels.[11] However, this quest to understand another's feeling is really an approximation. According to Martin and Hanington, practicing designers may use short-term flexible approaches to approximate the full immersive experience.[12]

One such example of the short immersive experience is The Sleepover Project, originally developed by David Dillard, president at D2 Architects. This project asks designers to spend 12 hours living in a senior living center, while engaging in empathic modeling strategies such as taping fingers to simulate arthritis, and then to document in a systematic method the experience in a journal.[13] They then use the journal and analysis to inform their practice. Although not nearly as immersive in time and length as MASS Design's Butaro Hospital nor Patricia Moore's study, the idea is for the designers is to better understand another's circumstances. These examples of empathic modeling highlight that stretching ones' empathic horizon can spur or unearth innovative approaches to solving problems, leading to new ideas and pushing the creativity that design teams see as valuable for making effective decisions.

New Perspective

Techniques that help the designer to gain a new perspective require stepping back out of the users' shoes and often involve engaging the users in co-design or participatory design strategies. Sometimes, the users may even take the lead, moving the designer to a facilitator's role. Doing so provides the users empowerment and ownership. In this process, it is important to acknowledge that you are not the same as the other. Designing *for* a client/user as opposed to *with* a client/user suggests a process of one party serving another. However, when empathy is at the center of the design process, a true partnership should occur. Ownership through participation in the design process on the part of the client/user helps to assure that the designs explore insights that meet the users' real needs.

Participatory design engages the different stakeholders, such as users or clients, in the design process for their contributions as experts. Such co-design is practiced in many diverse ways. It may be used as an independent discipline or as part of methodologies in other areas of practice with varying degrees of user engagement. Such methods range from vocal leadership involvement of users in a workshop in the design process to physically building of a prototype to demonstrate their skills in realizing their ideas. The common goal of all methods is to better understand the users' experience through the users' participation or even their leadership. According to Sanders, participatory design allows the designer to view users, consumers, or customers as experts who understand their own ways of living and working.[14]

This relationship contrasts with user-centered design, which although user focused, positions the designer as the expert advising the user who consequently serves just as a representative. Rather, participatory design is a more human-centered design approach that values and respects the users for their contribution.

The higher the value that the designers place on the users'"expertise" by engaging them in the design process, the more they will gain understanding of the users and their emotions and experience. An example of participatory design in practice that effectively asked users to not only contribute to the design process, but enabled them to lead the design and development of their community is the Ibasho

Café Project. It started in Ofunato-City, Japan, in February 2012. After the Great East Japan Earthquake in 2011 resulted in many displaced communities, a team from the nonprofit Ibasho organization visited Ofunato and conducted interviews with elderly survivors who, a year after the disaster, were still living in temporary housing. By starting out as problem seekers on a quest to understand context, the team members were impressed by the tales of heroism and gratitude the community expressed, despite horrific loss. However, they quickly realized that the conversations with the community members revealed something stronger—a deep desire by the elders to help rebuild their communities. Yet, the community was uncertain how to accomplish this. An opportunity arose for the team to help guide, but not direct, this community in their quest.[15] During an 18-month span, Ibasho organized at least ten community workshops. In these workshops, Ibasho elders led community members of all ages to develop a shared vision of the purpose, design, and operations of the café. This meant challenging preconceived notions about the appropriate role for elders.[16]

Beyond contributing their ideas within the early workshops, the elders were engaged with the construction decisions (see Figure 12.1).

The design shows a dedication to the organization's mission to trust the elders in being the experts in understanding their own way of living to help guide the design process (see Figure 12.2).

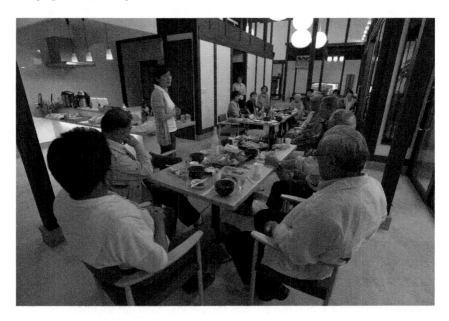

FIGURE 12.1   The Ibasho Café, which opened in June 2013, is not only a thriving café spot for the elders within the community to gather, but it serves as a place where the elders babysit for younger families, and employ younger community members to work within the café

Source: Courtesy of Ibasho

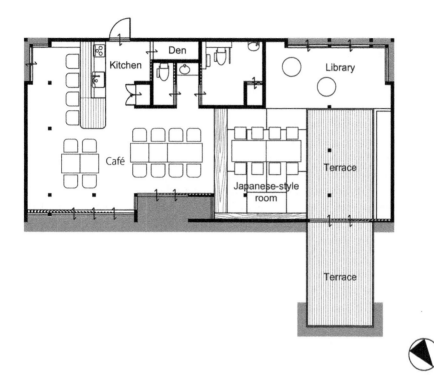

FIGURE 12.2   Plan of the Ibasho Café (Built from a traditional Japanese farmhouse that was deconstructed and relocated to the affected Massaki area)

Source: Courtesy of Ibasho

Participatory design or co-design activities are techniques employed to value the expertise and wisdom of older users, and have the potential for engaging younger users as experts in their way of living, particularly with school, museum, and hospital projects. Co-design activities, such as model making or building, can encourage children to explore by doing. However, often children are just as capable of participating in more structured traditional user-group meetings and can help to unearth problems not considered by other user groups. Unfortunately, often the design team does not bring children into the design process. This can result in missed opportunities to gain insight and understanding of their experience.

Despite the advantages of employing participatory design strategies with young and old user groups, definite perceived or real challenges exist. Just as with immersive research techniques, major hurdles to using participatory design techniques or co-design are time and resources. It takes time to collaborate and to be problem seekers, let alone problem solvers. Additionally, clients may not understand the value nor want to pay for the time. Furthermore, design teams need to have their own members instructed in how to facilitate participatory activities—so that they understand how to act as a partner with the users and not be tempted to take over and direct or lead.

Another major challenge to participatory design is failure of the design team to follow through with what they start. Because Ibasho engaged the elders from the start and valued them as experts, and then continued to respect their ideas throughout the entirety of the project, the Ibasho Café was a success. Otherwise, it might have been a post-disaster building relief effort by an outside organization that imposed its planning on a community. In other cases, where users are engaged as experts early on, but somewhere along the way, they are relegated back to being representatives, the project may not reflect the true values of the community. Designers need to be careful not to involve users only as a symbolic gesture for the sake of tokenism, as users may feel let down or marginalized.

According to Newman and Thomas, the danger when working with youth on school-design projects is that some participatory methods may promise more than they can deliver. This may result in unintended consequences.[17] If the plans of young people are rejected as too expensive, impractical, or unworkable, then the youth will feel discouraged and may disengage from both the process and conceivably from the educational system.

The scope of participatory design and its methods are quite expansive and used across many spectrums in the fields of design. It is critical that empathic designers step back, observe, and seek out an objective perspective after immersing themselves in the real world of the users.

The reality is that when the students participated in the design of the school study, there was the potential for as much risk for empowerment and positive outcomes as for disengagement. Students with varying learning levels were asked to participate in the co-designing activities. The gifted art students were requested to model ideas and create opportunities to lead and express their ideas through their expertise. However, what served equally or perhaps even more empowering was when the students from the special needs program began to lead as experts in their way of living and advised "the experts" on how the designs could be more inclusive.[18]

This example illustrates the idea that ownership is closely tied to empowerment. Empowerment by the user means that the designer has to let go and give ownership to the users, and has to let designs evolve beyond the designers' control. This can be destructive when designers are chasing what Dohr and Portillo[19] call the "idea of a 'perfect space.'" The best solutions require many conversations and revisions. The perfect space is not realized until the end user moves in and completes the process. Empowering users requires designers to let go of what they consider perfect. Thus, for empathy to be at the core of the design process, the designer needs to trust and let go.

Finding a Balance

Empathic design techniques of *stepping in* or *stepping back*, whether formal or informal, will reveal lessons for designers. Designers need to find a balance between the subjective and the objective, the aesthetic and the functional, the qualitative and the quantitative. As designers face increasingly complex project requirements, existing formal tools can help keep these competing variables in check. Pre- and post-occupancy evaluations can help reveal truths and opportunities for growth and performance.

A post-occupancy evaluation (POE) is a formal research strategy intended to evaluate and measure a built-design project's performance corresponding to the overall design objectives.[20] Design teams may use it as a tool for informing future projects by highlighting successes and lessons learned. With an increase in evidence-based design (EBD), tools such as a POE can help give guidance and structure to design decisions.

The Ibasho Café Project was part of a pre- and post-occupancy evaluation supported by the World Bank's Global Facility for Disaster Reduction and Recovery (GFDRR) to assess, as part of its Inclusive Community Resilience program, the effect of the Ibasho approach on Ofunato's (Japan) recovery.[21] Their 58-page document systematically provides a detailed overview of the project including its principles and design process, research methodology, and a synthesis of research findings, lessons learned, and research tools.

No matter the format being followed, it is important to develop early on in the design process a clear plan for considering both the intended use to be measured and the users. Without a clear direct plan, qualitative or quantitative data may be collected, but is neither valuable nor useful to the designers or to the various stakeholders.

Complicated project timelines, such as in community development or health care, can extend beyond the expected and original objectives; intents may change over time. Whether domestic or international projects, any set of variables can prolong timelines. Regulations with building issues or governmental bodies can further affect the schedule. Thus, despite early strategizing for identifying desired outcomes to be measured, long project schedules may necessitate instituting flexibility and adaptability with the research tools.

As discussed earlier, the Ibasho Café Project engaged the elders of the community in participatory design strategies. Team members facilitated workshops in planning and design and then immersed themselves as participant-observers within the community for a year after the building was occupied to assist in the conduct of interviews and the collection of survey data. The data helped identify lessons learned. Empathic design strategies were clearly at the heart of the Ibasho Café Project as demonstrated in several of the lessons learned; these included investing time in project goals and engagement of users in the design process. This led to empowerment of the elders and community members who could take the lead while the team stepped back.

As with all projects that seek to dig deep and engage empathic strategies, there are challenges to overcome. The team also learned that flexibility and adaptability are not just needed when addressing time and schedules. Pre-existing conflicts, part of the fabric of any community, can affect community-driven projects. These projects need to be given time to establish their own timetables to adapt and grow with the project.

The report identified an interesting lesson learned relating to ownership and the completion of the perfect space Dohr and Portillo described as really only occurring when the user occupies and makes the space theirs.[22] This includes decorating it or adjusting it as they use it. Set-aside funding allowed for adjustments—both cosmetic and functional—for when the space is open.[23] This requires building operational change into the design funding, which may seem unrealistic for most projects. Yet, it may be interesting to explore how designers can help owners address future-users' needs. The results from the GFDRR and the tools and techniques used to assess the Ibasho Café Project were shared publicly. They provide a clear path for growth and learning in the quest to reach the users at a deeper level.

Future

The recent discoveries within science regarding the importance of empathy to our society and the past writings about the healing properties of empathy help situate empathic design as a significant construct within design for health and well-being. Exploring as if we are in the shoes of another is an important part in helping to imagine the possibilities of innovation as we look to heal through design. Innovation in form and structure helps to drive the design forward. However, we need to continue to seek out opportunities for exploring a deeper connection to reach the users and their real needs as a catalyst for innovation.

Juhani Pallasmaa, in *Empathic Imagination: Formal and Experiential Projection*, suggests that we are designing experiences. Architecture is not just about geometry or aesthetics, but about affirming our existence and emotions as we interact with the material world.[24]

The future of empathic design will not only require the designer to rely on using empathy to help understand the individual human encounter, but it will involve a larger cultural shift. It will require moving beyond individuals to transform society. Van der Ryn suggested that this change will not only include a human-centered approach that considers the needs of others, but that this transformation will require changes that affect the broader society.[25] Whether it is in nature, institutions, behaviors, or relations, this change is the idea that these designs look to answer bigger questions within society than the building alone can answer.

Several of the projects discussed in this chapter demonstrate that we may be closer than we think to this type of transformation and power of design to increase creativity. Beyond stepping into the users' shoes, stepping out for reflection and learning, these projects demonstrate designers going further and systemically having an impact on their communities. Empathic strategies are true to a human-centered approach and embrace deep design thinking.

The Butaro Hospital Project by the MASS Design Group began as one project that increased economic opportunities for the region by training 2,000 locals to learn new skills. This opportunity grew to a partnership with the Rwandan government to build more hospitals. Now MASS has begun raising funds to construct the African Design Center—a pilot architecture and design school in Kigali,

Rwanda. The Ibasho Café of Ofunato, Japan, developed as one project, has morphed into an organization that spurs creativity. After the Ibasho Café Project was completed in Ofunato, money was provided for a peer-to-peer exchange between elder community members of Ofunato and elders in Ormoc in Leyte, Philippines, devastated by Typhoon Haiyan in November 2013. Elders from both communities shared views on the disasters and their recovery experiences. More importantly, they swapped ideas on how elders of both communities can contribute to strengthening community resilience. The transformation shows an empathic process, guided by the users.

Conclusion

As we look to the future, it is important to understand the users who we are engaging and for whom we are designing. We also need to address what effects innovation in design and its effect on emotions and experiences. Time, money, and attitudes can all get in the way of employing empathic strategies. Yet, if learning and growing are to take center stage, we must bring empathy into the design process and not be overcome by the obstacles.

Notes

1 Sim Van der Ryn, *Design for an Empathic World Reconnecting to People, Nature, and Self* (Washington, DC: Island Press, 2013), 33.
2 Tara Mullaney, Helena Pettersson, Tufve Nyholm, and Erik Stolterman, "Thinking Beyond the Cure: A Case for Human-Centered Design in Cancer Care," *International Journal of Design* 6, no. 3 (2012): 29, www.ijdesign.org/ojs/index.php/IJDesign/article/view/1076/525.
3 David Howe, *Empathy: What It Is and Why It Matters* (New York: Palgrave MacMillan, 2012), 177.
4 Roman Krznaric, *Empathy: Why It Matters, and How to Get It* (New York: Penguin Random House Group, 2014).
5 Merlijn Kouprie and Froukje Sleeswijk Visser, "A Framework for Empathy in Design: Stepping Into and Out of the User's Life," *The Journal of Engineering Design* 20, no. 5 (2009): 437–448.
6 Howe, *Empathy*, 177.
7 Dorothy Leonard and Jeffrey F. Rayport, "Spark Innovation Through Empathic Design," *Harvard Business Review* (November–December 1997): 102–113, https://hbr.org/1997/11/spark-innovation-through-empathic-design.
8 Joyce Thomas and Deana McDonagh, "Empathic Design: Research Strategies," *The Australasian Medical Journal* 6, no. 1 (2013): 1–6, http://doi.org/10.4066/AMJ.2013.1575, www.ncbi.nlm.nih.gov/pmc/articles/PMC3575059/pdf/AMJ-06-01.pdf.
9 Roger Coleman, Cherie Lebbon, and Jeremy Myerson, "Design and Empathy," in *Inclusive Design: Design for the Whole Population*, eds. John Clarkson, Roger Coleman, Simeon Keates, and Cherie Lebbon (London, UK: Springer-Verlag, 2003), 482.
10 Marika Shioiri-Clark, *TEDxStellenbosch-Marika Shioiri-Clark Empathic Architecture* [Video file], August 2011, www.youtube.com/watch?v=KTXqJ2fZ0gA.
11 Jon Kolko, *Well Designed: How to Use Empathy to Create Products People Love* (Boston, MA: Harvard Business Review Press, 2014), 75.

12 Bella Martin and Bruce Hanington, *Universal Methods of Design: 100 Ways to Research Complex Problems, Develop Innovative Ideas, and Design Effective Solutions* (Beverly, MA: Rockport Publishers, 2012), 124.

13 Rodney Brooks, "Architects Live in Senior Living Space to Help Elderly," *USA Today*, August 2014, www.usatoday.com/story/money/personalfinance/2014/05/18/seniors-retirement-assisted-living/8006755/.

14 Elizabeth B. N. Sanders, "Perspectives on Participation in Design," 2013, 61–75, www.maketools.com/articles-papers/Sanders2013Perspectives.pdf.

15 Emi Kyota, Yasuhiro Tanaka, Margaret Arnold, and Daniel Aldrich, *Elders Leading the Way to Resilience, Global Facility for Disaster Reduction and Recovery* (The World Bank, 2015), 16, www.gfdrr.org/sites/default/files/publication/Elders-Leading-the-Way-to-Resilience.pdf.

16 Ibid.

17 Michelle Newman and Peter Thomas, "Student Participation in School Design: One School's Approach to Student Engagement in the BSF Process," *CoDesign* 4, no. 4 (2008): 246.

18 Ibid., 244.

19 Joy Dohr and Margaret Portillo, *Design Thinking for Interiors: Inquiry, Experience, Impact* (Hoboken, NJ: John Wiley & Sons, Inc., 2011), 121.

20 Sally Augustin and Cindy Coleman, *The Designer's Guide to Doing Research* (Hoboken, NJ: John Wiley & Sons, Inc., 2012), 255.

21 Kyota, Tanaka, Arnold, and Aldrich, *Elders Leading the Way,* https://www.gfdrr.org/sites/gfdrr/files/.../Elders-Leading-the-Way-to-Resilience.pdfreference.

22 Joy Dohr and Margaret Portillo, *Design Thinking for Interiors: Inquiry, Experience, Impact* (Hoboken, NJ: John Wiley & Sons, Inc., 2011), 121.

23 Kyota, Tanaka, Arnold, and Aldrich, *Elders Leading the Way*, 30.

24 Juhani Pallasmaa, *Empathic Imagination: Formal and Experiential Projection 2014*, 82.

25 Van der Ryn, *Design for an Empathic World.*

13

THE ROLE OF PLACE IN WELL-BEING

Lisa Waxman

Introduction

Our lives are influenced and shaped by the places we have lived and the people we have met along the way. There are places that tug at our hearts, places we dream about, and those we long to revisit. In *Lure of the Local*, Lippard reflects on the human need for a place to stand and for something to hang on to.[1] Places ground us, to the earth, to the communities in which we live, and to each other. Places provide a starting point, the opportunity to belong somewhere, and a place to return to. The value of "place" in our lives cannot be underestimated.

There are people who are fortunate to have places that provide comfort, roots, and a stability that grounds them. Much of this comfort is stored up in memories created over a lifetime—all which are tied to the places in which living has occurred. I have vivid memories of my early childhood in Shrewsbury, Massachusetts, and our dead-end street where many kickball games and snowball fights took place. There was winter sledding on the "big hill" at the elementary school and we stayed out until our toes were numb and the sun began to set. Then we moved to Tallahassee, Florida, and that comfort was upended—for a while at least. Until we settled in a new neighborhood full of children who also liked kickball, flashlight tag, and evenings filled with touch football games. In both cases, neighbors knew and supported one another—it was safe and there was comfort in the certainty of our lives.

I was lucky to have a childhood set in wonderful places that provided a strong sense of community. However, for others, their story of place looks very different. For the homeless, to whom all spaces are temporary, or for foster kids who bounce from family to family, the special places that ground so many other lives may never be theirs. Older adults who must leave their homes in order to be cared for elsewhere leave a lifetime of memories behind. Refugees may flee their homes seeking a safe haven from civil war and violence. Other families may lose homes to natural disasters such as fire, hurricanes, or earthquakes. In all these cases, special places were left behind and the losses are real and profound.

A professional colleague recently shared his own loss of place. Years ago, he had purchased an old house in San Diego and rebuilt it doing much of the work with his own hands. There were blood, sweat, and tears, as well as a significant amount of money invested in the property. Ten years later he had to sell the house for financial reasons. He explained, "That house was a grounding force for me, and I have yet to find the same sense of stability and security."

This chapter will address the value of place in solidifying wellness and well-being in our lives. To fully explore the concept of place in this context, the meanings underlying our association with place will be examined. This will be followed by a discussion of social capital, the value of connection with those in our communities, and place attachment, the bond of people to places. The chapter will conclude with a list of design recommendations that can help designers create meaningful places.

The Meaning of Place

We live, work, and play, as well as give birth, receive an education, meet new friends, build careers, recover from illness, and grow old in places shaped by designers. These places become enriched with memories and the meanings we attach to them. Meaning making, as it relates to place, is a part of everyday life and helps us create order from chaos and uncertainty. We make sense of our world by reflecting on what is around us and synthesizing it with what we already know and believe.

Sometimes the meaning attached to space is the result of long-accepted truths—referred to as *a priori* assumptions—with meaning derived from reason.[2] Conversely, meaning can be constructed based on experiences—a more subjective way of knowing that is unique to an individual's personal experiences. This way of knowing, referred to as *a posteriori*, is meaningful and trustworthy to those involved in the process. Making meaning this way is the basis of the constructivist approach to creating knowledge, which is grounded in the situations in which it occurs combined with what the individual brings to the experience.

Place experiences begin with a person and a place, their interpretations of that place, followed by their subsequent behavior and the memories and meaning that become linked with the experience. Spaces are experienced in the moment, and in a slice of time, all set within a social context.[3] Lefebvre emphasizes the importance of the system of individuals and objects that occupy space and the process of constructing, destroying, and reconstructing the space again and again over time.[4] Moore writes that the process by which we come to know the environment is an active one that is mediated by our continually evolving experiences.[5] Our perception of place can be viewed as part of an active search for meaning.

Social Capital and Our Need for Place

The United States is a mobile society, teeming with people on the go search-ing for the next adventure or opportunity. For many, mobility is associated with development, personal growth, and open-mindedness, while a lack of mobility may represent parochialism and restricted opportunities.[6] In this same vein, the United States is a country that prides itself on pervasive busyness with people reporting being too busy or working too hard.[7] With so much movement, what happens to the human need to pause, make connections with others, and develop a bond to the place they live?

Research tells us that despite our tendency towards mobility, many individuals express a desire to live in a connected community with opportunities for social networking.[8] In *Bowling Alone*, Robert Putnam investigates the collapse and revival of the American community and explores the many variables that strengthen or weaken the bonds of a community.[9] Putnam refers to these bonds as *social capital*, which he defines as the connections among individuals that create social networks, thereby laying the groundwork for mutual trust and support.[10] When social capital is present, generalized reciprocity is expected—which means, I'll do for you and expect you will do for me at some point in the future if I need you. Communities with strong social capital look out for fellow neighbors and are more likely to come together in times of need.

The presence of social connections in a community has many benefits, includ-ing positive influences on health and happiness.[11] Generally speaking, being part of a social network contributes to one's sense of purpose, feelings of belonging, sense of security, as well as the impression of self-worth, which can result in greater motivation for self-care along with a modulation of stress.[12] Social connections are important because they give rise to the perception that in times of hardship, one can rely on others for support.[13] The opportunity to depend on others has been shown to enhance a person's ability to cope with demands, thereby lowering the impact of stressful situations.[14] In addition to mediating stress, when people are more integrated with others in their communities, they are less likely to experience heart attacks and cancer, and infant mortality rates are lower.[15] The social influence of fellow community members also provides access to normative guidance regard-ing health-related behaviors, such as exercise or smoking.

When social capital is present in a community, the benefits to public spaces are many. Public spaces are typically cleaner and well cared for, people are more likely to be friendly, and neighborhoods are safer.[16] Jane Jacobs found that when cities are designed to increase contact among neighbors living in the community, people feel safer and are more likely to stay put in their community.[17]

There are many factors that impact the presence of, or lack of, social capital, including the existence of places in which connections and relationships can be cultivated. Interior designers, architects, landscape architects, urban and regional planners, and others involved in the design of the built environment, all play a part in creating the places in which opportunities for social connections with others are made possible. The location, design, staffing, and culture of a place shape the activities that happen there and the clientele who gather. Gathering places in a community evolve throughout the years as society changes and different building types and gathering spaces emerge.[18] The role of place cannot be overemphasized in community building.

Place Attachment

When people talk about communities they love, they often speak about the places that make those communities special. Whether it is natural spaces, public parks, restaurants, retail establishments, or family homes, those places are an essential part of what makes the community stand out. Over 20 years ago, Setha Low and Irwin Altman defined the term place attachment as the bonding of people to places.[19] This bonding, connection, and feeling of rootedness that develops when people are attached to places are important factors in overall human well-being. Scannell and Gifford found that ties with people, groups, objects, and places are essential to connect people with their environment, as well as their past and their future.[20]

David Seamon suggests that place is a factor in the creation of "lifeworlds", which involves the daily routines of people in places and the meaning that is attached to those experiences.[21] Seamon explains that "places hold lifeworlds together and provide a center from which people define human meaning and intention that helps establish place".[22] He sees people moving through the world in a sort of "place ballet" where daily routines are intertwined in time and space. These everyday ballets between people and place create the frameworks with which place attachment is formed. Attachment to place can be sustained and even strengthened by the recurrence of these routines.

Ray Oldenburg writes about the "third place", those places that are not our home, and not our workplace, but the places in which "people happily collect in informal gatherings outside of home and work".[23] He defines third places as those that are neutral ground, welcome people from all walks of life, and provide opportunities for conversation. They typically have clients who are regular patrons, a playful atmosphere, and are not necessarily in locations or buildings that are high profile—meaning they may not impress the uninitiated at first glance. These spaces serve as a home away from home, and in some cases, can even compete with home.

Good design creates places in which people can gather, formally or informally, in either planned or unplanned encounters, with others who may become good friends, casual acquaintances, or simply familiar strangers. Friendships are often formed with people with whom we share common interests or values. However, the presence of casual acquaintances in the places we inhabit has value in that it provides opportunities to let others into our lives.[24] People are circling in the same orbits, sharing the same lifeworld, and are linked as members of the same community. Most importantly, they are known to each other. These casual associations should not be undervalued as they enrich our lives and help ground us within a society.

When Spaces Become Places

When planning the design of a space, a designer seeks to understand how the space will be used and what features are necessary for it to function in a way that meets the client's needs. These needs may include spatial allocations, circulation and adjacencies, technological needs, sustainability considerations, and potential adaptations for future use. However, well-trained designers are also interested in what can be done to make the space a "place", and carefully explore what that means to each project and each group of end-users. Taking a space and elevating it to the level of "place" may happen accidentally, but it is more often the result of careful planning on the part of the designer. Creating places takes sensitivity on the part of the designer that looks at functional needs, but also how the space will feel and support the user.

Designing Places for Well-being

What makes a great place? There is no magic formula or recipe for the design of successful spaces. Furthermore, any recommendations should consider the uniqueness of each person, as well as the nuances of each locale and its climate, culture, and history. At the risk of over-generalizing, the next section of the chapter will synthesize research from many environment and behavior researchers and designers with the goal of creating guidelines for the design of spaces that have the potential to become places. A dozen recommendations will be presented below that can assist designers interested in more human-centered design.

Design Should Recognize Its Responsibility to Humankind

The ability to shape spaces as a designer is an enormous responsibility. The Interiors Declaration written by designers assembled by the International Federation of Interior Architects/Designers in 2011 outlines the value, relevance, responsibility, culture, business, knowledge, and identity of interior architects and interior designers.[25] The declaration emphasizes the value of design in establishing a sense of place, as well as a sense of who we are, and of what we can be. The declaration reminds us that great spaces are essential for a great culture and that spaces can help us learn, reflect, imagine, discover, and create. Designers must consider the needs of people—both health and safety, as well as their overall well-being. It emphasizes the value of design for humanity, the most important client, and the designer's responsibility in shaping the human experience.

Design Should Consider Its Purpose

Even the most attractive designs lose their luster if they don't work for their intended purposes. Designers should remember they are designing places where life events are experienced. Listening to the client and end-users regarding how they will use the space, what they hope to accomplish in the space, as well as how they would like the space to feel, are important considerations. In addition to listening, a designer should use evidence-based design research to inform decisions. Research can help enlighten projects and lay the groundwork for a successful space.

Design Should Consider Location

Settings differ, not only in appearance, but also in factors impacted by the climate, culture, and the history of a locale. Good design should be informed by the past and by the geographic and historical contexts of its location. As globalization expands there is a greater chance of homogenization of places. Day questions designs that are built for one location and simply dropped into another without consideration for local nuances.[26] He explains that buildings may be placed anywhere, but may not belong. When considering location, one must also consider what is immediately adjacent to a space. Every space borders something, whether it is an open field, a high-rise building, a public park, or any number of other spaces. The same is true of interior spaces where there is interplay between spaces adjacent to one another. Consideration for the location and adjacencies results in a better, more human-centered design.

Design Should Provide a Sense of Order

Typically, humans prefer environments where there is a sense of order—especially when spaces are not familiar.[27] In their environmental preference framework, Kaplan and Kaplan include legibility, which focuses on the ability to make sense of a space.[28] Lynch's elements of legibility include paths, edges, districts, nodes, and landmarks— features of a space that help lend order to an environment.[29] Order can be brought to a space in many ways, but often includes navigation tools and points of reference that help people know where they are. Spaces should be intuitive to users and communicate by providing cues as spaces are navigated. Furthermore, visual harmony can produce a sense of order when spaces are assembled in ways that avoid confusion. Generally speaking, order can be produced when spaces are clearly organized and people have a sense of where they are.

Design Should Respond to Human Imprint

Places are successful when they allow people to alter spaces so they work and feel right. People should sense that a space welcomes adaptations that make it more user-friendly. There is no behavior apart from the environment in which it takes place. When design sends a message that it is unyielding, people may hesitate to adapt the environment to better accommodate their needs—even if that environment is oppressive. Sommer calls this "hard architecture", which occurs when spaces resist human imprint. However, spaces that allow individuals to alter their surroundings allow the control that so many people desire.[30]

Design Should Provide Opportunities for Human Connection

Designers have a responsibility to think about how a space will serve the human need for connecting with others. These connections are greatly influenced by the proximity of people to one another as well as the paths they take. Deasy emphasizes the importance of designing to encourage friendship formation by considering features such as stairs and walkways arranged so users can have space for casual encounters with others.[31] Connections can also be enhanced by providing welcoming, user-friendly lobbies, cafés, break rooms, and other spaces where people can engage with one another. Generally speaking, design that makes chance encounters with others in a person's "life orbit" possible enhances the user experience.

Design Should Allow For Privacy, Territoriality, and Control

These three aspects of human behavior are closely related. Privacy allows people to control access to them, whether it is spatial, visual, auditory, or informational.[32] Privacy provides opportunities for solitude, self-reflection, and control over information communicated about oneself. With territoriality, spaces can be claimed on a short-term basis (a lunch table) or on a more permanent basis (a work office).[33] Both access to privacy and the ability to establish a territory provide more control to users. Generally speaking, people prefer to have control of their surroundings and the ability to adapt them to meet their needs.

Design Should Wisely Use Resources

If design is to contribute to human well-being then smart, sustainable decisions should be made that use the earth's resources wisely. Conducting thorough research on products to examine their impact on the environment is essential to making smart, sustainable decisions. Designers should also consider the human cost of resources. What are the labor conditions involved in harvesting, extraction, production, and shipping of a product? Are resources exploited in areas of the world where people are powerless to stop it? The challenge for designers is to make habitable spaces that leave a healthy and habitable world for generations in the future.

Design Should Support Human Health and Well-being

Health and well-being, as it relates to design, can be examined on many levels. People spend up to 90 percent of their time indoors, thus the quality of the interior environment is essential to health. Selecting materials that greatly reduce or eliminate indoor air pollution creates healthy air quality that contributes to occupant well-being. It is also important to mention health and fitness and how a building's design can positively impact users by encouraging movement. On a larger scale, neighborhood walkability can positively impact all people, especially as concern grows over increasing obesity rates. Consideration for quality lighting, access to daylight and views, as well as good thermal and acoustical comfort also contributes to health and well-being.

Design Should Be Authentic

How can authenticity be put into the practice of design? As mentioned earlier, good design should be attentive to the climate, culture, and the history of a space. Vernacular architecture and design—the architecture and design of the locale—helps create an identity for people who live in a community. Honesty in materials, which has been a point of discussion in architecture and design for many years, comes into play when discussing authenticity. With material honesty, wood is used as wood, metal as metal, ceramic as ceramic, etc., and materials are represented as what they are. Over time, material honesty has become more complex as materials and products have become more advanced. In many cases, new materials have the potential to make buildings perform more efficiently. Perhaps the answer is to let each user have their own experience and determine if it is real and authentic to them.

Design Should Restore

At some point, everyone needs an opportunity to rest and restore. There are many ways an environment can create opportunities for restoration. Lighting and access to views are essential components of a pleasing environment with the potential to restore. Access to nature has been shown to have a positive impact on restoration as well. Stephen and Rachel Kaplan developed the Attention Restoration Theory, which focuses on the attention required in a given situation, and how that impacts our ability to restore and recharge.[34] Nature has been shown to be very effective in providing opportunities for a restorative experience. When designers bring nature into a space, provide views, natural light, or easy access to outdoor spaces, users have the opportunity for restorative experiences.

Design Should Be Adaptable

Buildings are typically designed with a specific user or group of users in mind. As people occupy the space, minor modifications are made to meet various needs. However, over time buildings often see major modifications or renovations to serve different users. Design doesn't stop when buildings are complete, but rather it is revised when occupied and adapted over time as needs change. These changes may cause feelings of dislocation, or people may learn to adapt.[35] Spaces should be designed with the future in mind and consideration of what a space may become.

Conclusion

There is power in design. Well-designed spaces should center us and provide a place to ground our everyday experiences. Designers have a responsibility to foster human experiences that are pleasurable and improve the quality of life. Good places should have a spirit and nourish those who spend time there through their beauty, function, and support of human needs. When places serve as a grounding force, we are able to go out into the world braver, more confident, and more inspired in our lives.

Notes

1 Lucy Lippard, *The Lure of the Local: Senses of Place in a Multicentered Society* (New York: The New Press, 1997), 27.
2 Dan O'Brien, *An Introduction to the Theory of Knowledge* (Cambridge, UK: Polity Press, 2006), 25.
3 Tiiu Vaikla-Poldma and Drew Vasilevich, "Poststructuralism, Phenomenology and Lived Experience: About Meaning Held Within Design and Spaces," in *Meanings of Designed Spaces*, ed. Tiiu Vaikla-Poldma (New York: Fairchild Books, 2013), 104.
4 Henri Lefebvre, *The Production of Space* (Cambridge, MA: Blackwell, 1995), 108.
5 Gary Moore, "The Development of Environmental Knowledge: An Overview of an Interactional-Constructivist Theory and Some Data on Within-Individual Development Variations," in *Psychology and the Built Environment*, eds. David Canter and Terence Lee (London: Architectural Press, 1974), 193.
6 Maria Lewicka, "On the Varieties of People's Relationships With Place: Hummon's Typology Revisited," *Environment and Behavior* 43, no. 5 (2011): 704.
7 Robert Putnam, *Bowling Alone: The Collapse and Revival of American Community* (New York: Touchstone, 2000), 189.
8 Alison Gilchrist, "The Well-Connected Community: Networking to the Edge of Chaos," *Community Development Journal* 35, no. 3 (2000): 264.
9 Putnam, *Bowling Alone*, 189.
10 Ibid., 19.
11 Sheldon Cohen, "Social Relationships and Health," *American Psychologist* 59, no. 8 (2004): 682.
12 Sheldon Cohen, Lynn Underwood, and Benjamin Gottlieb, *Social Support Measurement and Intervention: A Guide for Social Scientists* (New York: Oxford University Press, 2000), 10.
13 Sheldon Cohen, "Psychosocial Models of the Role of Social Support in Etiology of Physical Disease," *Health Psychology* 7, no. 3 (1988): 285.
14 Sheldon Cohen and Thomas Wills, "Stress, Social Support, and the Buffering Hypothesis," *Psychological Bulletin* 98, no. 2 (1985): 347.
15 Ichiro Kawachi and Lisa Berkman, "Social Cohesion, Social Capital, and Health," in *Social Epidemiology*, eds. Lisa Berkman and Ichiro Kawachi (New York: Oxford University Press, 2000), 181.
16 Putnam, *Bowling Alone*, 307.
17 Jane Jacobs, *The Death and Life of Great American Cities* (New York: Random House, 961), 333.
18 Clare Cooper-Marcus and Carolyn Francis, *People Places: Design Guidelines for Urban Open Space* (New York: John Wiley & Sons, 1998), 1.
19 Setha Low and Irwin Altman, "Place Attachment: A Conceptual Inquiry," in *Place Attachment*, eds. Irwin Altman and Setha Low (New York: Plenum Press, 1992), 4.
20 Leila Scannell and Robert Gifford, "Comparing Theories of Interpersonal and Place Attachment," in *Place Attachment: Advances in Theory, Methods, and Applications*, eds. Lynne Manzo and Patrick Devine-Wright (New York: Routledge, 2014), 23.
21 Dave Seamon, "Architecture, Place, and Phenomenology: Buildings as Lifeworlds, Atmospheres, and Environmental Wholes," final draft, www.academia.edu/14128043/Architecture_Place_and_Phenomenology_Buildings_as_Lifeworlds_Atmospheres_and_Environmental_Wholes_forthcoming_2017_.

22 David Seamon, "Place Attachment and Phenomenology," in *Place Attachment: Advances in Theory, Methods, and Applications*, eds. Lynne Manzo and Patrick Devine-Wright (New York: Routledge, 2014), 12.

23 Ray Oldenburg, *The Great Good Place* (New York: Marlowe & Company, 1989), 16.

24 Lisa Waxman, "The Coffee Shop: Social and Physical Factors Influencing Place Attachment," *Journal of Interior Design* 31, no. 3 (2006): 48.

25 "IFI Interiors Declaration," *International Federation of Interior Architects/Designers*, wwwifiworld.org.

26 Christopher Day, *Places of the Soul* (Burlington, MA: Elsevier Press, 2002), 13.

27 Roberto Rengel, *Shaping Interior Space* (New York: Fairchild, 2007), 9.

28 Stephen Kaplan and Rachel Kaplan, *Cognition and Environment: Functioning in an Uncertain World* (New York: Praeger, 1982), 86.

29 Kevin Lynch, *The Image of the City* (Cambridge, MA: MIT Press, 1960), 47.

30 Robert Sommer, *Tight Spaces: Hard Architecture and How to Humanize It* (Englewood Cliffs, NJ: Prentice-Hall, 1974), 1.

31 Cornelius Deasy, *Designing Places for People* (New York: Whitney Library of Design, 1985), 18.

32 Julie Stewart-Pollack and Rosemary Menconi, *Designing for Privacy and Related Needs* (New York: Fairchild Publications, 2005), 1.

33 Deasy, *Designing Places for People*, 18.

34 Rachel Kaplan and Stephen Kaplan, *The Experience of Nature: A Psychological Perspective* (Cambridge: Cambridge University Press, 1989), 177.

35 Vaikla-Poldma and Vasilevich, "Poststructuralism, Phenomenology and Lived Experience," 102.

14

DESIGNING FOR SPIRITUALITY

Jill Pable

Introduction

Human spirituality is an interesting and, at times, provocative topic. Deeply embraced by many through religious or other expressions and scorned by others, people's perspectives on the subject are remarkable in their variety. The connections between spirituality and its manifestation in built architecture are only now being considered in a more holistic way.

This chapter will review literature from both empirical and artistic camps, which are growing in unison. Spirituality not only matters, but is also highly underestimated in its ability to provide grounding and orientation to the lived human experience. Further, sacred architecture is an important means by which to promote that spiritual sense through its ability to act as a bridge between the tangible and ethereal.

Context: The Current State of Western Culture

A deeper discussion of the built space's role in spiritual wellness should begin with a review of spirituality itself. Does spirituality matter in today's age, and if so, why? To ask this question in the beginning of the twenty-first century is particularly interesting, given the degree of change that currently affects daily life on many fronts. New York Times editorial writer David Brooks identifies the current age as one of general unrest, ignorance and disdain for the spiritual aspects of life.[1] There is both direct and indirect evidence for this conclusion.

Children often live in chaotic environments without guidance or stable living arrangements. In the United States, a first-world country, 22 percent of children live in poverty, and 45 percent live in households classified as low-income.[2]

Communities possess few social bonds or boundaries for behavior, likely because they lack a system of standards of how to relate to each other. A growing division of wealth, political and racial distinctions has likely exacerbated clashes in Ferguson, Missouri, Dallas, Texas, and other locations.[3]

Natural resources are increasingly a catalyst for want, disagreement and even war. Disregard for the earth's health has rendered some cities' air quality inhospitable, and led Pope Francis to release the Vatican encyclical publication *Laudato Si': On care of our common home*, which links unchecked human activity and spiritual disconnection to these choices of waste and pollution.[4]

As people seek to maintain required separation of their spiritual aspects from daily life in a democratic society, schools do not, and cannot, acknowledge spirituality for fear they are proselytizing.[5]

Further evidence for the decline of spiritual prioritization in the West comes from a recent Pew Research Center survey that assesses peoples' spiritual attitudes within the United States.[6] This report discusses the rise of the 'nones'—those citizens that indicate, when asked their religious preferences on surveys, that they are unaffiliated (and also includes agnostic, atheist and other designations). While reasons are not empirically confirmed, the politicization of religion by conservative factions and the millennial generation's general disengagement from belonging to organized groups are considered factors in this change.[7] No matter what the cause, these trends are of concern to some, as they may indicate the emergence of an adult cohort that lack the spiritual vocabulary to reason and ground actions in thoughtful context.[8]

Despite the decreasing trajectory in religious affinity evident in these indicators, different evidence points to an enduring need for human beings to maintain a sense of meaning and positivity in their lives:

- The self-improvement knowledge industry is a 9.6 billion dollar market replete with motivational speakers, books, seminars, retreats, institutes and personal coaches.[9]
- With its easy means to make friends and share details of life with like-minded people, social media is an outlet for spiritual engagement and improvement. Spiritual leader Deepak Chopra has 1.2 million followers on Twitter across the globe.[10]
- Western society is experimenting with new belief systems ranging from Feng Shui to the Jewish mystic belief of Kaballah, Christian Science, and Scientology. The Mormon religion has existed only since 1830, yet now has more members than the Jewish faith.[11]
- While far from positive, extremist movements that link themselves to religious beliefs find followers in those that seek to 'right' the world by adherence to a chosen set of religious edicts.

In summation, cultural trends paint a picture of a world hungry for meaning and purpose that bring order from chaos. Whether people embrace religion or not, national polls consistently show that spiritual matters are a concern to a large majority of Americans.[12] This stance echoes the Pew Research Institute's recent findings that of those Americans that state they have no religious affiliation, more than a third said they nonetheless value spirituality.[13]

Spirituality Defined

While people vary in their acceptance and desire to develop their spiritual dimension, spirituality as a topic is not well understood. The nineteenth century American

religious philosopher and psychologist William James has offered a succinct definition of spirituality in *The Varieties of Religious Experience*, describing that spirituality
is a belief that an unobservable order exists.[14] Dyson, Cobb and Forman's literature review concludes that spirituality addresses the human need for transcendence
beyond ordinary experience and embodies a connection to others and the self.[15]
These experiences are processed individually, and they are difficult to convey due
to the limits of how people communicate.

When reviewed comprehensively, these definitions converge around three main
ideas:

Belief in order, or an underlying logic and possibly intention of things
A connection to oneself and others
The need for transcendence, or a view beyond current observable life

This chapter will discuss these themes, first from the perspective of empirical science, and then through the lens of architectural theory.

Spirituality and Religion are Related, But Different

For the layperson, being 'spiritually oriented' and 'religious' may be seen as the same
thing. However, for many writers on the topic, there is a distinction between these two
concepts, with spirituality as a sort of 'ticket in' that permits one to then embrace a
specific religious view. One well-known proponent is Christian apologist and Oxford
scholar C. S. Lewis. In *Mere Christianity* Lewis explains the logic of belief—not in
Christianity specifically, but instead in a bedrock sense of spirituality characterized
by gut level sense of right and wrong.[16] For example, a person may feel wronged by
another who takes 'their' seat in a room they had vacated only for a moment. Lewis
describes that the disagreement between the two people progresses along the lines of
defending their action by conformance to a commonly held but undefined rule of law
(the seat didn't appear to be claimed, so it was fair play to take it). Both people subscribe to this same unwritten code of 'fair play'. Seldom, however, does the argument
circle around the notion that the two people hold different fundamental standards.
Thus, Lewis suggests that 'decent' behavior and more broadly, morality, is universal,
and this code espouses traits common to most religions such as generosity, kindness,
courage, honesty and truthfulness. For Lewis, then, spirituality is an underlayment for a
religious affiliation that one can then actively choose to guide one's life choices.

Empirical Evidence for a Human Spirituality
and Wellness Connection

A relatively new perspective on the definition of spirituality and its distinction
from religious affiliation comes from the emerging voice of empirical scientists
from fields including psychology and neuroscience. There is a growing consensus of
spirituality as a phenomenon with an observable, provable genetic component that
everyone possesses. Religion, in contrast, entirely springs from one's conditioning
environment. Spirituality can, but does not have to, include religious expression.

What does it mean to have spirituality in one's life? What is the worth of a transcendent foundation? Until recently, these questions went largely unexplored within empirical sciences. Considered unapproachable from a measurement perspective, a spiritual worldview was considered exclusively a matter of faith and belief.[17] However, new findings are starting to challenge these pre-assumptions, compelling the hard sciences to make a case for the objective utility of a developed spiritual sense.

Within the last 15 years, a body of credible and verifiable research has been published in recognized research journals that examines spirituality and its effects on human systems. These works from biology, psychology, medicine, physics and neuroscience have been recently analyzed by Columbia University psychology researcher and fellow of the American Psychological Association Lisa Miller in several works including *The Oxford Handbook of Psychology and Spirituality* (2012) and more recently *The Spiritual Child* (2015). Miller outlines several general findings about spirituality that are beginning to coalesce within researchers' findings.

Innate and Present From Birth

People experience spirituality through a biologically grounded capability present from birth. This instinct is as present and vital as one's physical senses, emotions and general character, and this innate need can either be supported or repressed through a person's lived social, psychological and physical environment.[18] One potential outlet for this spiritual capability is religious participation. While there is not yet universal agreement on this point, Miller argues that unlike other childhood characteristics that emerge and radically evolve, a primal spirituality 'antenna' is present within a person from early on, preceding even language acquisition. This is evidenced by children's cultural-transcendent instinct to act in ways that are spiritually motivated—for example, to give, to be inquisitive and to wonder about life's puzzlements such as bears, stars, grasshoppers and clouds.

While children may be attuned to spiritual influences by nature, other things can affect the extent of a child's engagement with this sense. Studies conducted on twins by Kendler, Gardner and Prescott suggest that the strength of a child's spiritual awareness is approximately 29 percent due to broad genetic heritability, 24 percent due to family environment and 47 percent due to a person's unique individual environment.[19] Approximately 30 percent of a person's 'antenna strength' for spiritual connection is due to genetics.

The desire for spiritual development may also vary throughout a person's life. Miller et al. have identified that spiritual awareness surges in adolescence, which is synchronous with the onset of depression for some individuals—and is something that spiritual assets can aid in counteracting.[20]

Spiritual Need and Effects Are Measurable, and Therefore Knowable and Verifiable

Empirical scientists are exploring the outcomes of people's adherence to spiritual beliefs. In one study, for example, adolescents with a strong sense of connection to a sense of transcendence were found to be 70 to 80 percent less likely to engage in heavy substance abuse and less likely to take sexual risks. Among teenage girls, having a strong spiritual sense was notably protective against serious depression.[21] Some young adults that lack this sense of spirituality fill the resulting void with gang affiliation, drug use or other forms of escapism. However, adults who consider themselves highly spiritual by the age of 26 are 75 percent more protected against recurrence of depression.

Other researchers, including medical doctors Cloninger, Svrakic and Przybeck have examined the state known as transcendence, often defined as identifying with a unified reality.[22] These researchers concluded that transcendent thinking is associated with physically detectable structural differences in the occipital and parietal regions of the brain. This structure is in turn associated with heightened levels of the neurotransmitters serotonin and dopamine, which can assist people to feel good about themselves. Neurologically speaking, there is still much to be learned about transcendent thinking, but some suspect that this thinking mode can compel the brain to 'get out of the way' or defer to higher tasks, turning down the volume knob on immediate cares and distractions, allowing attendance to other matters.

Spiritual Orientation Affects More Than One's Mental State

The studies that Miller has reviewed examine spirituality's influence on people from diverse empirical science approaches.[23] What has emerged is that not only are the benefits of spirituality significant and measurable, there is also a common physiology that underlies mental states such as depression and transcendence, confidence, identity and other significant issues. Given spirituality's ability to act as a sort of compass, then, it is not surprising that this foundation sense also unites the brain and body, affecting a person's thinking *and* actions.[24] Spiritual connection is in touch with one's core of individuation, deeply affecting people's foundation perceptions of life, including:

their approach to the world
sense of meaning and purpose in the world
nature of one's deepest self
approach to work and relationships
understanding of reality
choosing right and wrong actions

If this influence of spiritual sense is valid, then it follows that a well-nurtured spiritual instinct may lead to actions that affect oneself as well as others and the community. For example, spiritual orientation and attunement can contribute to the civility of society as evidenced by the extent of criminality, sense of community, and, more broadly, a culture's collective progress toward its future.

Three Dimensions of Human Spirituality from Empirical Science

Fifteen years of inquiry by empirical scientists has yielded a beginning definition of spirituality. A further, more specific set of findings also has begun to clarify three distinct dimensions of human spirituality.[25] These are helpful to the purpose of this chapter because they provide a list of needs within the human psyche to which architecture and design might respond.

Natural Spirituality

'Natural spirituality' refers to the innate, present-from-birth spirituality capacity discussed above. Existing alongside other human qualities such as consciousness, the physical senses, the intellect and emotional qualities, this biological-based faculty can be harnessed by people at their option to achieve transcendence, either through religious beliefs and actions or other means.[26]

Relational Spirituality

Human beings often experience transcendence by communing with others. This could be other human beings and/or another higher power. In this way, relational spirituality is closely akin to bonding and human love.

Heart Knowing

'Heart knowing' is the least directly verified, but commonly observed in clinical studies conducted on people engaged in meditation. A loose definition of this concept is an intuitive knowledge about being a part of a larger entity or universe. This transcendent feeling varies from sensing a relationship with God to having an affinity with nature or an inner wisdom.[27]

A Potential Place for Architecture amongst Spirituality Empirical Findings

With a brief discussion of spirituality in light of empirical science concluded, this discussion now turns to spirituality as expressed through physical architecture. What real or potential role does the built environment play in helping people achieve transcendence and cultivate their spiritual dimension? Obviously, intentional and unintentional places of worship that set the stage for transcendent thinking have been constructed from the earliest human history, such as the caves of Lascaux, gothic cathedrals, Zen gardens, Egyptian pyramids, Aztec temples and today's churches, to name but a few. To consider the place of built environment in a person's quest for spiritual development is to start to mix the world of matter with the world of intangible thought, and more generally to comingle artistry with science. The proper approach to this endeavor as scientific, artistic or something in between has perplexed thought leaders for some time.

There may be some agreement for the thought that architecture has a significant role to play in transcendent thinking formation from the empirical science camp as well. In the Kendler et al. study referenced previously, researchers determined that the capacity for a person's propensity for deep spiritual connection is *47 percent due to a unique personal environment.*[28] While these researchers do not specifically call out the influence of buildings and places in this lattermost category, it is logical to include one's physical surroundings in 'personal environment', and intriguing to see the potential role that tangible places might play in promoting a transcendent ability, especially with the benefits this can bring to peace of mind and thoughtful action. Miller's conclusions from her review of empirical studies adds credence to this potential for spiritual architecture, identifying that the natural capacity for a transcendent relationship can be cultivated for some people through beauty, nature and reflection—all elements that architecture can introduce or support in the human experience.[29]

The Nature and Impact of Sacred Spaces from an Architectural Perspective

The potential contribution of architecture to achieve a state of transcendence may have support from empirical science, as suggested above. If such connections exist, then the long-standing fascination held by both the public and architectural designers with transcendent places may have utility beyond what instinctual aesthetic intentions have lent up until now. Architectural critique and commentary have long described architectural projects whose design decisions were prompted by the desire to impart deep meaning in churches, mosques, chapels and other spiritually oriented, secular projects.[30,31,32,33] Indeed, critics and essayists in architecture have eloquently defined architecture's role as inseparable from meaning and spirituality, defining the spaces as a means to integrate worlds that were formerly disconnected.[34,35] In sacred texts themselves, that path to enlightenment is often told in architectural terms that can include bridges and gates.[36] For architectural theorist Thomas Barrie, architecture gives place to needed ritual, and without this suitable setting, such traditions risk being meaningless.[37]

Barrie's Framework of Meaning in Sacred Architecture

With architecture's connection to spirituality thus introduced, this chapter next examines a framework for meaning in spiritual architecture so that a comparison of it to empirical science's findings on spirituality can be made. Architect and theorist Thomas Barrie has examined, personally visited and photographed spiritual spaces from many of the world's faiths. He concluded that meaning in sacred architecture occurs in three ways that use tangible elements manipulated by designers.[38] First, 'site' encompasses those aspects of a sacred place that impart meaning in an explicit and detailed way. Stained glass of pictorial scenes in a Christian church is an example.

Second, Barrie identifies that sacred places provide needed settings for rituals and ceremonies, and in this way support a sense of community among believers. The torii arches of the Shinto religion, for example, demarcate the distinction between secular and sacred space, and declare the increasingly holy nature of space as they repeat themselves along the path to worship.

Third, Barrie identified that form is a conveyor of meaning in a way that is more abstract than 'site'. For the Muslim believer, the Ka'aba signifies the House of God through its geometric purity and is the central element around which pilgrims must walk seven times on the *hajj*. Barrie's primary point is that spiritual architecture operates at a series of levels of comprehension and consciousness for its human users, which simultaneously opens avenues for tangible expression for architectural designers and expands the opportunity for connection for its recipients.

Parallels between Empirical Science Findings and a Spiritual Architecture Framework

While Barrie's framework is worthy of note in its own right, its details are also interesting when examined alongside conclusions about human spirituality currently emerging from empirical science. Table 14.1 juxtaposes the two three-part frameworks of human spirituality when examined both from empirical science findings discussed earlier in this chapter by Miller[39] and Barrie's three aspects of architectural meaning in sacred spaces.[40]

A close consideration of these two very different approaches in understanding the nature and preferred expressions of human spirituality show interesting parallel conclusions. Their similarities reveal a potential alignment of scientific findings of neurology, biology and psychology determined through positivist experimentation and the design-through-instinct approach that has long been an architectural tradition. For example, Miller's 'natural spirituality' is mirrored in Barrie's celebration of the natural site as a foundation from which to experience transcendence—both are pre-existing. Second, Miller's relational spirituality has an associative doppelganger in Barrie's acknowledgement of architecture as an oft-necessary setting for these ceremonies,

TABLE 14.1 Comparison of Three-Part Frameworks for Human Spirituality from Empirical Science and Architecture

Aspects of human spirituality from empirical science	Natural spirituality: an inborn, innate sense of spiritual connection that transcends culture, geography	Relational spirituality: experience of transcendence through relationships with other human beings, with ourselves, or a higher power	Heart knowing: perception of the sacred through inner wisdom, a transcendent sense, or through the body
Barrie's three levels of human meaning that occur in sacred architecture	The natural (given) and built site (architecture) present a fundamental platform from which to experience transcendence	Rituals and ceremonies occur, and architecture acts as a stage that accommodates and facilitates myth transferal, teaching, and discussion	Architecture facilitates meaning at a deeper, abstract level within the composition of form, which can occur at the subconscious level

Sources: Data from Miller (2015); Barrie (1996).

reinforcing the importance of communal connection both in empirical evidence of human beings' fundamental needs and their architectural settings. Lastly, both frameworks give credence to the notion of deep, subconscious levels of spiritual engagement with heart knowing and architectural form. This last point, the least defined in the hard sciences, is arguably one of the most compelling aspects of architecture.

A Sacred Architecture Example, Interpreted Through The Conjoined Science/Architecture Framework

Given that two complex frameworks are the focus here, it is helpful to explore how these three aspects of spirituality and sacred architecture might be expressed within an actual completed project. An intriguing subject for this exercise is the 9/11 Memorial Museum in lower Manhattan, New York City, and is arguably an intensely spiritual, yet secular space. Each of the three parts of the combined framework considered in Table 14.1 is here considered.

Natural Spirituality (Science): Natural and Built Site (Architecture)

There is emerging scientific evidence that humans empathize with the sorrow of others, according to researchers that examined fundamental neurophysiological functioning.[41] The 9/11 Memorial Museum presents a tangible architectural platform from which to experience the grief of this large-scale event. Geographically positioned right on top of one of the focal locations for this terrible tragedy, the case could be made that locating it elsewhere would have reduced its meaning and impact. See Figure 14.1.

Relational Spirituality (Science): Rituals and Ceremonies (Architecture)

Emerging scientific consensus declares that transcendence (and the psychological and physiological benefits that come with it) can be nurtured through relationships with other people, oneself or with a higher power.[42] The grieving process often involves a sense of communal camaraderie. In the 9/11 Memorial Museum, the exhibits form the setting for shared conversations of loss and meaning through individual perusal, or interpretive tours hosted by docents that encourage personal connection, accommodating collective remembrance so that the tragedy's lessons can be retained by future generations.

Heart Knowing (Science): Form on the Subconscious Level

Clinical evidence suggests that there is a deep level to spiritual understanding that does not always rise to the level of conscious awareness. Architecturally, the 9/11 Memorial Museum's architectural design emphasizes its natural site impact by drawing visitors down into a hollow in the earth where the Twin Towers once stood, promoting a powerful confrontation of the psyche with meaningful physical

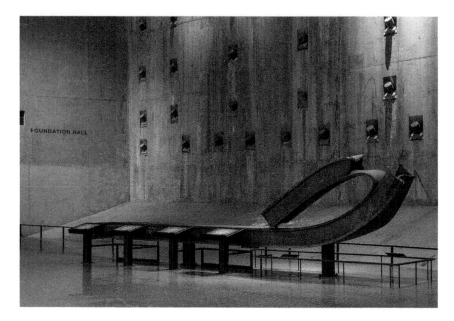

FIGURE 14.1 The tremendous scale of the destruction is made clear by world trade towers structural steel beams bent double. In the Museum's context, they become visually powerful teaching tools infused with meaning.

Source: Photograph by Jin S. Lee, 9/11 Memorial Museum

space. Architecturally, the designers of the 9/11 Memorial Museum tap tactics of volumetric pressure and release as well as harness the element of contrast, phenomena that the typical visitors may not notice in and of themselves, but are likely calibrated to deeply resonate with emotional effect. See Figure 14.2.

Implications

It is striking that two organizational frameworks about how people engage and are affected by spirituality emanated from two very different viewpoints—one from observable scientific discovery and the other from instinctual architectural precepts, and both have arrived at many of the same conclusions. There are several potential implications in this convergence: First, science is now confirming what those that desire transcendent spaces and their designer-builders have known for a long time—in a gut instinct sort of way. This may imply that architectural designers and builders through time have reacted to what naturally is most meaningful to their human users. It is only recently that science is confirming these architectural hunches and feelings, but science is taking it a step further by verifying physical and psychological benefits for people that have embraced their spiritual side. In his book *Proust was a Neuroscientist*, Jonah Lehrer describes other instances where art in fact led science in confirming the veracity of an idea for human improvement.[43]

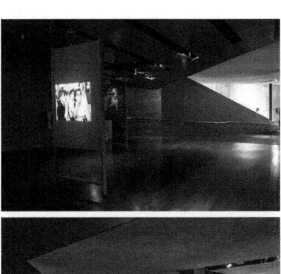

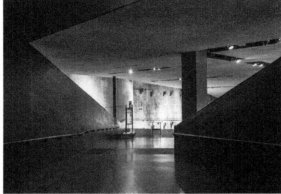

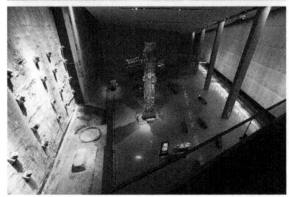

FIGURE 14.2 This image series captures the unfolding visitor experience near the museum's entrance. The intentional dark squeezing of space is punctuated by eyewitness audio and video stories, subtly implying deep despair. This leads the visitor to the illuminated balcony, which reveals the deep pit in which the Twin Towers' remaining slurry wall serves as a remaining witness and logical form giver.

Source: Photographs by Jin S. Lee (top and middle) and Amy Dreher (bottom); Included by permission of the 9/11 Memorial Museum

Second, the alignment of these two sets of findings, and the implication that architecture may play a verifiable role in accommodating psychological and biologically-based spiritual needs may underscore the uniquely suitable role (and perhaps responsibility) architecture plays in assisting people to become fully actualized and capable of transcendence.

So what of the intersection of spirituality, wellness and architectural space? A review of emerging empirical consensus when viewed alongside architectural theory on sacred space suggests that these three concepts are critically important to human actualization, and all are likely linked to each other. Perhaps when people arrive at similar conclusions from very different beginning points of knowing, there is a better chance that things are so. This view of reality and its potential relationships assigns to designers the full responsibility as shapers not only of space, but also of thought, and makes them significant influencers of the future. On this, empirical science and aesthetic reasoning appear to agree.

Notes

1 David Brooks, "The Next Culture War," *New York Times*, August 4, 2015.
2 National Center for Children in Poverty, "Child Poverty," National Center for Children in Poverty, www.nccp.org/topis/childpoverty.html.
3 Suzanne McGee, "Protests Over Michael Brown's Death in Ferguson Show America's Struggle With Inequality," www.theguardian.com/money/us-money-blog/2014/aug/19/race-ferguson-inequality-opportunities-african-american-injustice.
4 Pope Francis, *Laudato Si': On Care for Our Common Home* (Vatican City, Italy: Libreria Editrice Vaticana, 2015), 17.
5 David Brooks, "Building Spiritual Capital," *New York Times*, May 22, 2015.
6 Pew Research Center, "America's Changing Religious Landscape," Pew Research Center, www.pewforum.org/2015/05/12/americas-changing-religious-landscape/.
7 Pew Research Center, "'Nones' on the Rise," www.pewforum.org/2012/10/09/nones-on-the-rise/.
8 Brooks, "The Next Culture War."
9 PR Newswire, "The Market for Self-Improvement Products & Services," www.prnewswire.com/news-releases/the-market-for-self-improvement-products--services-289121641.html.
10 Neha Prakash, "Deepak Chopra: Spirituality in the Age of Social Media," http://mashable.com/2012/09/17/deepak-chopra-spirituality-social-media/.
11 Pew Research Center, "America's Changing Religious Landscape."
12 Tom Barrie, Julio Bermudez, Anat Geva, and Randall Teal, "Architecture, Culture & Spirituality (ACS) Creating a Forum for Scholarship and Discussion of Spirituality and Meaning in the Built Environment," Architecture, Culture & Spirituality, www.acsforum.org/history.htm.
13 Pew Research Center, "'Nones' on the Rise."
14 William James, *The Varieties of Religious Experience: A Study in Human Nature* (Gutenberg Project, 2014), 53.
15 Jane M. Dyson, Mark Cobb, and Dawn Forman, "The Meaning of Spirituality," *Journal of Advanced Nursing* 26 (1997): 1183.
16 C. S. Lewis, *Mere Christianity* (San Francisco, CA: Harper Collins, 1952), 18.
17 Lisa Miller, *The Spiritual Child: The New Science on Parenting for Health and Lifelong Thriving* (New York: St. Martin's Press, 2015), 51.
18 Miller, *The Spiritual Child*, 53.

19 Kenneth S. Kendler, Charles O. Gardner, and Carol A. Prescott, "Religion, Psychopathology and Substance Use and Abuse: A Multimeasure, Genetic-Epidemiologic Study," *American Journal of Psychiatry* 154, no. 3 (1997): 325.

20 Lisa Miller, C. Tenke Wickramaratne, and M. Weissman, "Religiosity and Major Depression in Adults at High Risk: A Ten-Year Prospective Study," *American Journal of Psychiatry* 169, no. 1 (2012): 93.

21 Alethea Desrosiers and Lisa Miller, "Relational Spirituality and Depression in Adolescent Girls," *Journal of Clinical Psychology* 66, no. 10 (1997): 1021.

22 C. Robert Cloninger, Dragan Svrakic, and Thomas B. Przybeck, "A Psychobiological Model of Temperament and Character," *Archives of General Psychiatry* 50 (1993): 981.

23 Miller, *The Spiritual Child*, 51.

24 Ibid., 40.

25 Ibid., 51.

26 Ibid., 53.

27 Ken Wilber, *Integral Spirituality: A Startling New Role for Religion in the Modern and Postmodern World* (Boston, MA: Shambhala Publications, 2006).

28 Kenneth S. Kendler, Charles O. Gardner, and Carol A. Prescott, "Religion, Psychopathology, and Substance Use," 325.

29 Miller, *The Spiritual Child*, 57.

30 Anthony Lawlor, *The Temple in the House* (New York: G.P. Putnam's Sons, 1994), 5.

31 Spiro Kostof, *A History of Architecture: Settings and Rituals* (New York: Oxford University Press, 1985), 18.

32 Thomas Barrie, *The Sacred In-Between: The Mediating Roles of Architecture* (New York: Routledge, 2010), 1.

33 Robert Birch and Brian Sinclair, "Spirituality in Place: Building Connections Between Architecture, Design, and Spiritual Experience," *ARCC Conference Repository*, 84, www.arcc-journal.org/index.php/repository/article/view/116/88.

34 Thomas Barrie, *Spiritual Path, Sacred Place Myth, Rithal and Meaning in Architecture* (Boston, MA: Shambhala, 1996), 7.

35 Lawlor, *The Temple in the House*, 5.

36 Barrie, *The Sacred In-Between*, 1.

37 Barrie, *Spiritual Path, Sacred Place Myth, Rithal and Meaning in Architecture*, 54.

38 Ibid., 5.

39 Miller, *The Spiritual Child*, 51.

40 Barrie, *Spiritual Path, Sacred Place Myth, Rithal and Meaning in Architecture*, 5.

41 Paul Hastings, Jonas Miller, Sarah Kahle, and Carolyn Zahn-Waxler, "The Neurobiological Bases of Empathic Concern for Others," in *Handbook of Moral Development* (New York: Psychology Press, 1986), 411.

42 Miller, *The Spiritual Child*, 72.

43 Jonah Lehrer, *Proust Was a Neuroscientist* (San Francisco, CA: Harper Collins, 2008), 57.

15

SAFETY, SECURITY, AND WELL-BEING WITHIN THE DIMENSIONS OF HEALTH CARE

Migette L. Kaup

Introduction

Health care is a complex system of programs, policies, and places. While designers are often focused more on the "place" part of the system, rather than the medical practices and health care policies, they should understand the entirety of the health care system in order to plan a truly comprehensive environment. This includes considering the experiences of health care delivery from various perspectives and the many ways that health care is delivered. Knowing more about these different viewpoints can afford designers the capacity to offset some of the negative "side-effects" deeply embedded within the practice of health care that may actually create barriers for individuals to be active participants in their own care.

When designing a setting intended to deliver care or support wellness, it is important to question whose interests are served. Architectural solutions can reveal a genuine philosophical view about the nature of human behavior and assumptions about what people are and what they need. This can be problematic as it often involves passing judgment on the lives and behaviors of ordinary people as well as a desire to reform them[1] if it is does not match the values of the health care provider. Gone unacknowledged, this approach may unintentionally drive some users away from the very services that are intended to help them.

All types of health care settings and what they are meant to accomplish are defined by a philosophy or a model of care and are understood by the set of goals that are realized organizationally, socially, and architecturally.[2] Therefore, this chapter will discuss health care as a system of supports that address the totality of what is possible when individuals are empowered to access information and make informed choices that are under their direction. The goal for designers is to understand the context of the health care settings and those cultural and psychosocial factors that influence how users will interpret the experience of those spaces. The potential of design to support the interactions between the patient and the provider in ways that empower people to be active participants in their own health and well-being will be explored.

Expanding Our View on Health, Safety, and Welfare in Design

Interior design professionals (in the United States and Canada) are obligated by professional standards to protect the "health, safety, and welfare" of the people for whom they design.[3] These expectations are enforceable through compliance with codes, standards, and regulations that protect human life. In health care design projects, designers are attentive to material specifications that can reduce the transmission of infections to help keep patients and providers "healthy." We can make sure that our designs are code compliant for egress in an event of an emergency to keep occupants "safe." And, we can apply accessibility criteria to spaces to enhance the autonomy and support the "welfare" of those who may have disabilities to navigate spaces. The scope of the obligation, however, goes beyond prescribed metrics of codes and regulations. Interior designers also have a responsibility to determine those psychological, cultural, and social considerations that will impact users and their experiences within the spaces they design.[4]

What if an individual doesn't "feel" safe in a setting because they perceive a threat to their cultural identity due to the visible features, symbols, and other sensory information that surround them? There are no prescribed standards for designing for these perceptual and cognitive experiences; it takes a deeper level of knowledge and inquiry on behalf of the designer to fully explore how to best meet diverse user needs. These variables may be increasingly complex and yet even more critical for groups who have had their sense of personal control stripped from them based on the assumed norms of other, more dominant groups. Therefore, designers must apply research-based skills to more fully understand different user perspectives.

In health care design, it is of utmost urgency that this understanding be developed as our global society is increasingly experiencing a disparity in access to even basic health services.[5] Those most vulnerable to not having equity in these environments include the young and the old, and individuals who identify with marginalized groups or under-represented minorities.

The Connection Between the Perception of Safety and Well-being

The perception of "being safe" comes from the ability to anticipate or predict the surrounding environmental conditions, and, to have a sense that others within that setting will not pose a threat. Feeling "safe" is also related to feeling "in control" and having the ability to manage the environmental situation. Feeling safe and being in control can have an exchanging dynamic when individuals are navigating a situation where they may encounter, or anticipate they will encounter, threats to their sense of self or be limited in their ability to control the situation.[6]

The inability to control stressful conditions may cause people to develop feelings of helplessness and to lose the determination to improve their circumstances.[7,8] The consequences of these types of encounters alone can result in poor health outcomes. Exposure to toxic situations (including fear and frustration) lead to a biological response that includes pathologic changes such as elevated blood pressure, stomach ulceration, shrinkage of lymphoid tissue, and enlargement of the adrenals.[9] If there is a persistent bundling, or layering of stressors across time, the more difficult it is for bodily systems to function optimally.[10] This break-down of human physiology has a negative impact on health and well-being in general.

Multiple studies over the years have demonstrated that there are measurable impacts on users that are related to environmental conditions.[11,12,13,14,15] When human action involves fear or anxiety, it can also interfere with the perceptual and cognitive processes. Designers can be instrumental in creating supportive settings that reduce the negative psychological effects of environmental stressors by considering how and when individuals can achieve personal control over these stressors through their behaviors, their cognitive appraisals, and their decision-making capacity.

Design of the System: Who's in "Control"?

Through the built environment, we create a backdrop for patterns of everyday life that are expected to be applied to all users of publically available settings. These spaces are designed around assumptions that the meanings and perceptual experiences will be similar because of the assumptions of shared norms.[16] In this manner, design has been a way for social control—a mechanism to direct action and influence agency. But whose sense of control is supposed to be enhanced in a health care setting? Through whose eyes is the designer looking when they are planning the spaces; the provider, or the receiver of care? Typically, designers do not get the opportunity to interact closely with multiple users of the space. They receive their information from those who are "in-charge" of providing the service. This means that the interpretation of the experience of that service and the spaces in which these services are delivered may miss important opportunities to convey a sense of inclusiveness.

Health care is a multi-faceted system designed to "control" information and "control" how individuals interact with care providers.[17] As a consequence the environment where health care is delivered plays a central role in communicating that the control is often one-sided.[18] The designer plays a central role in creating an experience that can convey a positive exchange between the patient and the provider, but in order to be effective in this role, they must understand the context under which various users may harbor fears and anxieties. Nine dimensions of experience can be used to consider the balance of control through place design.[19] The basic premise of these dimensions is to consider how built form and features of space can influence use and patterns of expected behaviors for individuals and between groups of people within a setting (see Box 15.1).

BOX 15.1 NINE EXPERIENTIAL DIMENSIONS OF PLACE THAT CAN INFLUENCE PERCEPTIONS OF CONTROL

Orientation/Disorientation: The design and configuration of spaces within a building can assist in orienting users, which empowers them to navigate the spaces independently, or, it can disorient users, which makes them dependent on others to find their way to their destinations.

Public/Privacy: Built from segments and organizes space in a manner that places certain kinds of people, places, and actions under conditions of surveillance while privileging other kinds of people, places, and actions in private conditions. This spatial segmentation mediates social encounters between people in ways that impact the control people have over their actions and the actions of others.

Segregation/Access: Boundaries and pathways can segregate places and therefore people by social status, gender, race, culture, class, and age, creating privileged enclaves of access to different amenities for different groups of people.

Social/Universal: Buildings are socially produced, which means that social "norms" of dominant groups drive the design standards. The result is that these design solutions are often presented as serving "everyone's" needs when in fact, they do not represent appropriate settings for the needs of under-represented groups who are still expected to use the spaces.

Stable/Change: Buildings often create a perception of permanence of place, a stable social order. This can be especially prevalent when buildings convey familiar cues or patterns that match social expectations. Different architectural forms and non-standard design features can, however, indicate a change in approach or process. This unfamiliarity can be unpredictable for some users.

Authentic/Fake: Material use in architecture and interiors conveys a strong indication of the substance of the place and the authenticity of the quality of the overall experience of space. Materials that convey an illusion of the properties of other materials, or materials that do not match the context of the settings may be perceived as foreign or unreliable.

Identity/Difference: Buildings and places inevitably convey meaning about the roles that people play in a setting and whether or not they belong. These messages are communicated through attributes and artifacts found in the setting as well as rituals regarding of the use of spaces.

Dominant/Subservient: Scale is an inherent factor in signifying power and control, and this scale can take many forms from the mass of a building and the volume of a space to the contents of items within spaces. The juxtaposition of large and small inherently signifies a relationship of power and may be linked to perceptions of domination and intimidation.

Place/Ideology: The experience of place has the capacity to move users deeply by the sensory and visual cues embedded in the setting. Yet, the very potency of place experience can render users particularly vulnerable to the ideological viewpoints of those who control these spaces.

Source: Framework adapted from Kim Dovey.

Design features emerge from these dimensions in ways that either enable or constrain human agency. These can be observed as we consider how the delivery of health care is enacted through the physical location where these services are provided and the details within the walls of these buildings. For example, health care setting are often full of physical symbols of authority (and control) institutionally embedded through rules and routines related to the use of the space from "check-in-desks" or nurses' stations, gated access to physicians, or icons and imagery of religious affiliations or corporate identities prominently placed throughout a facility (see Figure 15.1).

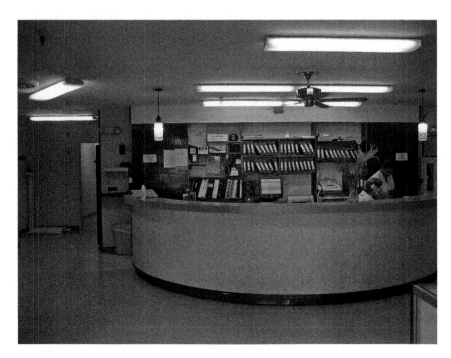

FIGURE 15.1   Nursing Stations Are Used as a Mechanism of Command and Control in Many Health Care Settings

Source: Photo by Migette L. Kaup

In order to better understand the perceptions of "safety" and "control" within health care, the unique needs of some under-represented groups are briefly explored and dimensions of control in the environment (as outlined in Box 15.1) are highlighted through examples. It is useful to understand different perspectives and social paradigms. When these narratives are effectively applied to decisions about place making, then the experiences of those spaces may be shaped in more positive ways for a broader range of users.

Designing a Safe and Supportive Health Care Environment for LGBT Users

One of our current social challenges continues to focus on the understanding and acceptance of diverse forms of gender and sexual identity. Individuals who identify as lesbian, gay, bisexual, or transgender (LGBT) have become an increasingly visible group who are advocating for deserved equality in the public (and private) domain. The litmus test of this equality is the civil right to have access to basic equality to goods, services, and places. LGBT individuals have unique experiences and unique challenges navigating health care services. Many of these individuals have grown up in homophobic and transphobic societies and have often encountered negative backlash associated with their gender or sexual identity.[20,21,22] Even if acts of aggression have not been experienced personally, individuals who have witnessed hostility towards groups with whom they identify may harbor feelings of insecurity in new environments and situations where they are uncertain of the reactions from others.[23] These fears and perceptions may be especially prevalent in older LGBT adults who have longer histories with discriminatory social and cultural forces.[24,25]

Some LGBT adults may not use health care services because they do not trust the *social environment* in which these services are delivered.[26] If they are "forced" to use them for critical care situations, as many as one in five LGBT individuals conceal their sexual orientation or gender identity from their physician because they do not perceive the potential interactions in these contexts to be emotionally supportive which can result in a negative quality of care.[27,28]

A 2015 study by Croghan, Moone, and Olson asked a large sample (n = 792) of LGBT baby boomers and older adults what they identified as the signals that convey a service provider is welcoming to diverse clientele and lifestyle needs. Responses from 327 individuals, who provided feedback on identifiable attributes, were analyzed and coded.[29] Final coding yielded 856 individual signal statements representing 44 codes.[30] Codes were then grouped into concepts of LGBT welcoming signals (see study for full report on individual concepts). While the results of this study should be carefully considered within the context of the limits of the sample (limited regional-base and age-range limitations of respondents), the outcomes point to some valuable indicators that designers and health care providers can use in their efforts to create an environment that is perceived to be "safe."

Social Versus Universal

Planning concepts focused on both verbal and non-verbal information consider the implications of presumed "*social norms*" versus more "*universal*" messages. Language and the use of terminology are significant. For example, discrimination, intentional or not, can begin with health and social service intake forms. Studies have shown that LGBT clients feel unsafe, uncomfortable, and disrespected when intake forms do not include diverse forms of marital status when identifying critical relationships and family support and/or gender and sexual identity.[31,32] Gender-based room identification, such as toilets, can also create stressful exchanges for individuals who identify with another gender.

Public Versus Privacy

The setting in which an individual is asked to disclose their health care needs may also contribute to fear of exposure of personal information. Privacy gradients within health care spaces should be carefully considered. Open reception areas that lack a sense of privacy discourage an authentic exchange of personal information when talking with staff. Clients who are already anxious about interactions with health care providers may feel stymied in their ability to safely convey their concerns or specific health care issues in settings with limited visual or acoustic privacy.

Identity Versus Difference

As an individual navigates an environment or situation, their perception and appraisal of threats will be shaped by multiple environmental cues and stimuli. Respondents noted that visual cues that convey a sense of welcoming, inclusiveness, and equity can include being selective in the choice and placement of imagery related to groups that are inclusive in their mission. An inclusive environment is more likely to limit overt cultural symbols that draw distinctions between groups. The designer's sensitivity to the nuances of features of a place can be instrumental in reducing the heightened sense of vulnerability for those who identify as LGBT.

"Out-Growing" the Space of Childhood: Supporting Adolescent Well-being

Moving from the stages of childhood into adult life is defined as the age of adolescence and can span from as young as 10 years of age to as old as 20 years.[33] This wide variance creates a gap in what is understood about approaches to care and the quality of that care for young adults due to the distinct developmental consideration that must be taken into account. It is commonly recognized, however, that young adults are often diminished or marginalized in participating actively in their health care choices.[34,35,36,37,38]

Kleinert outlines a host of issues that confront young adults around the world and many of these issues cut equally across socio-economic groups such as drug, tobacco, and alcohol misuse, sexually transmitted infections, obesity, eating disorders, or other nutritional challenges.[39] These factors create complex challenges for both health and overall well-being as this cohort experiences changes in emotional cognitive functioning that takes place during this stage of development.[40,41]

Fear is a common factor in preventing young people from getting either care or information they need.[42] These fear factors covered multiple domains—fear about lack of confidentiality and privacy, fear about being taken seriously or legitimately by adult providers, fear of being disrespected or acted upon without their consent.[43] Health systems are also entangled with strict controls and concerns about parental consent and may exacerbate situations or limit choices for addressing health care needs in the most appropriate manner.

Six groups of health care services settings have been identified as important in broadening access for adolescents.[44] Each may have unique nuances in their design attributes, and should be responsive to the particular goals of the health care services provided as well as responsive to the unique characteristics of young clientele (see Box 15.2).

Identity Versus Difference

The overall setting of the clinical atmosphere can set a tone for the occupants of the space. Infantile features, such as scaled down furniture and media and materials

---

BOX 15.2 SIX TYPES OF HEALTH CARE SERVICE SETTINGS DIRECTED AT THE NEEDS OF ADOLESCENTS

1. Hospital-based centers specializing in adolescent health and care. May be structured to accept walk-in appointments, or, may be structured to deal specifically with chronic care issues for young adults.
2. Community-based health facilities that might be a part of general practice or family-planning clinics.
3. Services that are integrated into school-based/college-based settings (resources close to other activities and services that are a part of the daily world of young people).
4. Community-based center that is a multi-service setting that offers other supportive resources and/or provides social and recreational activities (may have referrals to more formalized clinical settings).
5. Pharmacies and shops that sell health care products (such as birth control) but do not provide treatments.
6. Outreach programs where information is delivered where youth gather spontaneous or socially (e.g., street corners, shopping malls, clubs).

(Created by Migette L. Kaup)

in a waiting area that are below the development level of the youth reflect a lack of appreciation for the teens' rights to participate in their health care decisions from the moment the visit begins.[45] Adolescents relate better to stimulation that addresses their developmental stage of life. For example, they might enjoy a poster of a music group more than a poster of Winnie the Pooh. Health care for adolescents could apply more creative approaches and consider applying the types of technologies teens already interact with on a daily basis.

Segregation Versus Access

Adolescents' preferences for engaging in their own health care decisions will vary on a variety of personal factors.[46,47] Their developmental level, however, should not be used as an excuse to exclude youth from active roles, as is frequently the case.[48] Studies have explored the desires of adolescents to have more of a voice in their health care, especially when there are chronic or critical health conditions.[49,50] Adolescents often describe their consultations with doctors as *isolating* and dis-powering especially if they are excluded from the discussions. As teens get older they have more complex questions. As adult reasoning skills begin to develop in adolescents, a conflict begins to occur as teens seek access to answers to health care questions that they may not want to ask in front of other family members.

Dominant Versus Subservient

Settings should encourage consultation communication in a manner that equalizes the roles of the physician and the young patient. They want a choice and a sense of equality in terms of power relationships.[51] The settings where these interactions take place are central to the experiences for youth. For example, it is a different dynamic to sit across from a doctor who is behind a large desk in an office surrounded by medical literature and imagery of medical authority versus at a round table in a comfortable consultation room with ergonomically appropriate chairs. Likewise, if a physician would like to provide an opportunity for a private consultation with a young adult, there should be a combination of small consult rooms for doctor/patient discussions with waiting areas close by for parents or guardians.

Supporting a Culture of Person-centered Care for Older Adults

Another marginalized group within the health care system is those who are at the very later stages of life. Decline in functional health status and a depletion of financial resources will often relegate many frail (often female) elders to institutional care; care that will further reduce their sense of autonomy and self-efficacy. These settings are also often designed around the premise that elders are not "able" to participate in their care, and staff will oversee all of the elders' needs. This assumption ignores how design can empower frail adults to manage their own space, and the consequence makes them dependent upon staff. Environments that impose multiple forms of dependencies on elders unnecessarily exacerbate their condition.[52] If residents are physical restricted by the environment to engage in activities of daily living (ADLs) this can lead to behavioral dependencies as elders "learn" to be helpless and dependent.[53]

Orientation Versus Disorientation

Long-term care settings (aka nursing homes) are health care environments where people are expected to "live," and yet many of these settings continue to be patterned after hospital wards.[54,55]As a result of the scale of these spatial layouts, residents may be limited in their ability to navigate the setting independently due to long distanced and disorienting features. The interior details, fixtures, equipment, and other amenities often focus on the clinical tasks and ignore or diminish the importance of overall well-being and quality of life for those being cared for (see Figure 15.2). Long hallways in nursing homes are difficult to manage for many elders due to the distance between spaces and the poor quality of lighting that is visually and cognitively confusing.

Dominant Versus Subservient

But institutional definitions of "safety" can translate to the setting dominating residents and preventing them from having much real control of their actions.[56,57]Architectural features such as doors are a simple example of how a message of control and access can be experienced.[58] If a resident's bedroom door is located on a public hallway where all visitors to the facility are allowed to pass freely, how much control does an elder feel he or she has in regulating who is going to enter their personal space? Used effectively through spatial design and carefully integrated details, however, features such as door access can transfer this control back to residents.[59,60]

Ultimately, the goal of long-term care design should be to create a system of "interdependency" that enhances the quality of life for residents.[61,62] This approach focuses on the remaining capacity of frail elders and their abilities to participate fully in their lives and the decisions about their daily routines and care. This type of care requires changes on several dimensions as features of spaces should be conceived around the abilities of residents. For example, consider how different a design solution for a spa bathing room is likely to be if the program instructed the designer to plan a space where frail residents could *bathe themselves* with support from staff versus planning a space for staff to "give" a resident a bath. The features and amenities and the spatial composition of these two solutions is likely to create notably different experiences for the resident and impact their sense of control.

Public Versus Privacy

People living in long-term care settings want the same things that other people want: as much activity to one's taste as possible; freedom to do what they choose where and when they choose it; comfort and companionship with one's family and

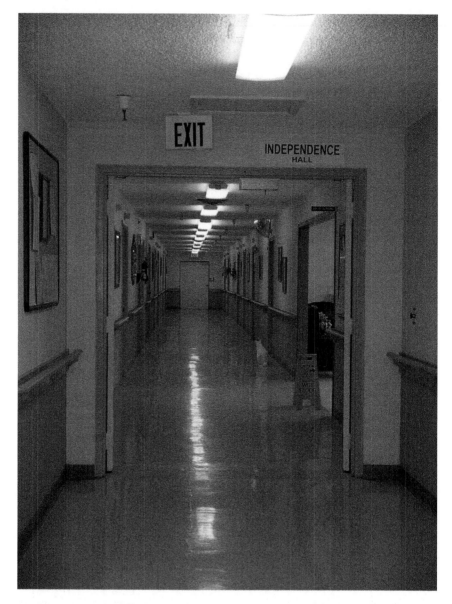

FIGURE 15.2 Long Hallway in a Nursing Home

Source: Photo by Migette L. Kaup

friends; and a safe environment.[63] Another dimension of institutional life, however, is the sacrifice of the type of privacy one would be afforded in their own home. Residents of long-term care still have need for intimacy in their lives and many are still sexually active. This reality is often ignored by care providers, families, and certainly by designers who think nothing of placing private bedrooms along public corridors. Design standards for resident rooms should be reconsidered in a manner that provides for and supports their autonomy, privacy, and dignity in a way that can actually be achieved through the space and amenities provided.[64] Even the simple furniture choices for the size of bed can have a significant impact on the ability of an elder to control their choices about intimate interactions.

Designers and long-term care providers should encourage and support continued research into the patterns of life and the routines that support overall well-being for elders in long-term care. We must continue to learn more about those aspects of the environmental milieu that create these experiences by equally engaging both theory and practice perspectives.[65] These approaches will provide the knowledge needed to plan long-term health care environments in a manner that will truly give residents autonomy and dignity.

Culturally Appropriate Design for Health Care in Remote Locations

Another group of individuals whose needs are not often understood includes those living in under-developed parts of the world and those displaced by conflict, ethnic wars, and other traumatic circumstances.[66] For these individuals, resources are extremely low, and accessing health care may require an extensive effort on their part. Designers must recognize how planning for health care services and spaces that support these services in areas may have unique dimensions.

Segregation or Access

Location and proximity to targeted groups is the first important consideration. Transportation to health care centers is a common issue for people living in rural areas.[67] Most individuals in under-developed parts of the world do not have access to personal vehicles and may have to travel long distances by foot just to access public transportation. In addition, terrain may also play a factor in both distance and time. Planning for health care centers in under-developed areas should, therefore, strive to bring health services closer to the communities. These peripheral health facilities can be instrumental in supporting medication maintenance, follow-up exams, and continuation of regular monitoring of health status which is vital for many who are being treated for HIV or other chronic conditions. These decentralized posts also have an opportunity to address primary care needs and the underlying determinants of health through the provision of pubic goods, such as water and sanitation systems.[68]

Place and Ideology

A common concern for groups living in remote areas is the distrust they have of outside others coming into their communities. Health care services are frequently provided by denominational groups and bring a religious frame of reference or ideologies that may not be shared with local cultures. Local spiritual leaders, medi-cine men and women, or other tribal elders may find these groups to threaten their status and authority, and as a result may discourage their followers from using these providers. In order for health care services in these communities to be effective and sustainable, planning and design efforts should engage a broad range of strategically identified stakeholders so solutions for needed services and the spaces they are delivered in respect and protect social and cultural rights.[69,70,71,72]

Public and Private

Researchers working with remote cultural groups note that the role of family in health care provisions must be carefully considered when planning not only the system of health care, but also when planning the nuances of these spaces. Based on familial structures and social expectations and norms, there may be very distinct needs for separation that must be considered within clearly defined spatial zones. For example, if a culture has strict expectations for separating genders, then entrances and the sequence of waiting and exam rooms may be dramatically impacted within the overall architectural layout. Likewise with expectations and cultural norms for circulation. Anthropometric and spatial criteria for design features may be influenced by ethnic characteristics as well as social and cultural norms inherent in behaviors and postures for different user groups. This can include such dimensions as stance, personal space boundaries, and gender roles. Some cultures and rural communities may not be accepting of a multi-story building that requires accessing spaces through the use of an elevator amongst their vernacular standard of ground level structures.

Authentic Versus Fake

Solutions must be culturally and contextually appropriate throughout all details of the setting. Designers who have only been trained in developed countries may be limited in their ability to incorporate features that respond to cultural context because they view them as counter to the health care standards to which they are accustomed. Rural clinics and health centers built with imported construction materials and technologies may, however, be less viable in the long-term. Extreme weather condi-tions, variations in use patterns, unreliable energy sources, and other environmental conditions will affect their life cycle in ways that are difficult to predict. Due to the practicalities of time and transportation, replacements may be difficult and a once modern facility may quickly be ineffective.[73,74] Designers and planning teams must understand the environmental situations that will be present in these communities and may need to consider a more vernacular approach to construction and design.

How to Move Forward

Health care is indeed complex, and user needs within a health care system are equally complex. A single set of design standards will not suffice, and planning and design cannot happen in a vacuum and effectively address the needs of patients or providers. Health care designers will continue to be challenged to learn how better to solve problems related to health and wellness in interdisciplinary teams and with experts from fields that may have little to do with medicine. They must also seek to work in innovative partnerships with low-income, nonprofit, and culturally diverse groups.

Expanding our cultural competencies in design should involve exploring the multiple environmental dimensions that contribute to health and well-being. Additional research is needed that more clearly contextualizes the health care setting and those cultural and socio-economic factors that influence the details of design.[75] The problems we confront will evolve with social history and shifting human behaviors that respond to the contextual situations around them.

We must remember that cultures are dynamic not static, therefore, we must continue to explore the changing dimensions of the narrative and lived experiences of the people who are served through our designs. How an individual identifies him/herself within a social structure is defined by multiple psychosocial variables. Designers should also remember that their assumptions about identity of marginalized groups are typically socially constructed based on the perceptions of meaning by others not a part of these groups. Today, we have a robust field of professionals who specialize in health care design. What they may lack is the background in cultural and social context that will allow them to more accurately translate their specialized design skills into meaningful places for extremely diverse sets of users. We must learn more to fully understand the diversity of human characteristics and how these characteristics and our wellness can be supported by design.

Notes

1 Simon Richards, *Architect Knows Best: Environmental Determinism in Architecture Culture From 1956 to the Present* (Ashgate Studies in Architecture, Farnham: Ashgate Publishing, 2012): 1.
2 Gerald D. Weisman, Habib Chaudhury, and Keith Diaz Moore, "Theory and Practice of Place: Toward and Integrative Model," in *The Many Dimensions of Aging*, eds. Robert L. Rubinstein, Miriam Moss, and Morton H. Kleban, (New York: Springer, 2000): 13.
3 Council for Interior Design Qualifications, "Definition of Interior Design," www.ncidqexam.org/about-interior-design/definition-of-interior-design/.
4 Council for Interior Design Qualifications, "Definition of Interior Design."
5 Ashley M. Fox and Benjamin Mason Meier, "Health as Freedom: Addressing Social Determinants of Global Health Inequities Through the Human Right to Development," *Bioethics* 23, no. 2 (2009): 112–122.
6 James S. Nairne, *Psychology: The Adaptive Mind* (Pacific Grove, CA: Brooks/Cole Publishing Co., 1997), 568.
7 Ibid., 563.
8 Ih Meyer, "Prejudice, Social Stress, and Mental Health in Lesbian, Gay, and Bisexual Populations: Conceptual Issues and Research Evidence," *Psychological Bulletin* 129, no. 5 (2003): 674–697.
9 Kenneth J. Thiel and Michael N. Dretsch, "The Basics of the Stress Response: A Historic Context and Introduction," in *The Handbook of Stress: Neuropsychological Effects on the Brain*, ed. Cheryl D. Conrad (Hoboken, GB: Wiley-Blackwell, Ltd., 2011): 3–28.

10 Leonard I. Pearlin, Scott Schieman, Elena M. Fazio, and Stephen C. Meersman, "Stress, Health, and the Life Course: Some Conceptual Perspectives," *Journal of Health and Social Behavior* 46 (2005): 214.

11 Roger Ulrich, Robert F. Simons, Barbara D. Losito, Evelyn Fiorito, Mark A. Miles, and Michael Zelson, "Stress Recovery During Exposure to Natural and Urban Environments," *Journal of Environmental Psychology* 11, no. 3 (1991): 201–230.

12 Charles J. Holahan, *Environmental Psychology* (New York: Random House, 1982).

13 Nairne, *Psychology: The Adaptive Mind.*

14 Shifra Sagy, "Moderating Factors Explaining Stress Reactions: Comparing Chronic-Without-Acute-Stress and Chronic-With-Acute-Stress Situations," *The Journal of Psychology* 136, no. 4 (2002): 407–419.

15 Thiel and Dretsch, "The Basics of the Stress Response."

16 Alan Wolfe, "Public and Private in Theory and Practice: Some Implications of an Uncertain Boundary," in *Public and Private in Thought and Practice: Perspectives on a Grand Dichotomy*, eds. Jeff Weintraub and Krishan Kumar (Chicago: University of Chicago Press, 1997), 196.

17 Diana J. Mason, "Family Presence: Evidence Versus Tradition," *American Journal of Critical Care: An Official Publication, American Association of Critical-Care Nurses* 12, no. 3 (2003): 190–192.

18 Mason, "Family Presence: Evidence Versus Tradition."

19 Kim Dovey, *Framing Places: Mediating Power in Built Form*, 2nd edition (New York: Routledge, Taylor & Francis Group, 2008), 18.

20 Karen I. Fredriksen-Goldsen, Charles P. Hoy-Ellis, Jayn Goldsen, Charles A. Emlet, and Nancy R. Hooyman, "Creating a Vision for the Future: Key Competencies and Strategies for Culturally Competent Practice With Lesbian, Gay, Bisexual, and Transgender (LGBT) Older Adults in the Health and Human Services," *Journal of Gerontological Social Work* 57, no. 2–4 (2014): 80–107.

21 Steve Gratwick, Lila J. Jihanian, Ian W. Holloway, Marisol Sanchez, and Kathleen Sullivan, "Social Work Practice With LGBT Seniors," *Journal of Gerontological Social Work* 57, no. 8 (2014): 889–907.

22 Meyer, "Prejudice, Social Stress, and Mental Health."

23 Ibid.

24 Fredriksen-Goldsen, et al., "Creating a Vision for the Future."

25 Meyer, "Prejudice, Social Stress, and Mental Health."

26 Gratwick, et al., "Social Work Practice With LGBT Seniors."

27 Fredriksen-Goldsen, et al., "Creating a Vision for the Future."

28 Gratwick,, et al., "Social Work Practice With LGBT Seniors," 890.

29 Catherine F. Croghan, Rajean P. Moone, and Andrea M. Olson, "Working With LGBT Baby Boomers and Older Adults: Factors That Signal a Welcoming Service Environment," *Journal of Gerontological Social Work* 58, no. 6 (2015): 637–651.

30 Ibid., 4.

31 Ibid.

32 Gratwick, et al., "Social Work Practice with LGBT Seniors."

33 Susan M. Sawyer, Sarah Drew, Michele S. Yeo, and Maria T. Britto, "Adolescents With a Chronic Condition: Challenges Living, Challenges Treating," *The Lancet* 369, no. 9571 (2007): 1481–1489.

34 Ibid.

35 Andre Tylee, Dagmar M. Haller, Tanya Graham, Rachel Churchill, and Lena A. Sa, "Youth-Friendly Primary-Care Services: How Are We Doing and What More Needs to Be Done?" *The Lancet* 369, no. 9572 (2007): 1565–1573.

36 Sabine Kleinert, "Adolescent Health: An Opportunity Not to Be Missed," *The Lancet* 369, no. 9567 (2007): 1057–1058.

37 Tanya L. Tivorsak, Maria T. Britto, Brenda K. Klostermann, Dawn M. Nebrig, and Gail B. Slap, "Are Pediatric Practice Settings Adolescent Friendly? An Exploration of Attitudes and Preferences," *Clinical Pediatrics* 43, no. 1 (2004): 55–61.

38 Bryony Beresford and Patricia Sloper, "Chronically Ill Adolescents' Experiences of Communicating with Doctors: A Qualitative Study," *Journal of Adolescent Health* 33, no. 3 (2003): 172–179.

39 Sabine Kleinert, "Adolescent Health: An Opportunity Not to Be Missed."

40 Tivorsak et al., "Are Pediatric Practice Settings Adolescent Friendly?"

41 Maria T. Britto, Robert F. Devellis, Richard W. Hornung, Gordon H. Defriese, Harry D. Atherton, and Gail B. Slap, "Health Care Preferences and Priorities of Adolescents With Chronic Illnesses," *Pediatrics* 114, no. 5 (2004): 1272–1280.

42 Tylee et al., "Youth-Friendly Primary-Care Services."

43 Ibid., 1566.

44 Ibid.

45 Tivorsak et al., "Are Pediatric Practice Settings Adolescent Friendly?"

46 Britto et al., "Health Care Preferences and Priorities," 1273.

47 Beresford and Sloper, "Chronically Ill Adolescents' Experiences."

48 Misha De Winter, Chris Baerveldt, and J. Kooistra, "Enabling Children: Participation as a New Perspective on Child-Health Promotion," *Child: Care, Health and Development* 25, no. 1 (1999): 15–23.

49 Beresford and Sloper, "Chronically Ill Adolescents' Experiences."

50 Ellen A. Lipstein, Kelly A. Muething, Cassandra M. Dodds, and Maria T. Britto, "I'm the One Taking It: Adolescent Participation in Chronic Disease Treatment Decisions," *Journal of Adolescent Health* 53, no. 2 (2013): 253–259.

51 Beresford and Sloper, "Chronically Ill Adolescents' Experiences," 177.

52 Wendy Lustbader, *Counting on Kindness: The Dilemma of Dependency* (New York: The Free Press, 1991).

53 Margret M. Baltes, "What Is Dependency?" in *The Many Faces of Dependency*, ed. Margret M. Baltes (New York: Cambridge University Press, 1996), 18.

54 Bruce C. Vladeck, "Unloving Care Revisited: The Persistence of Culture," in *Culture Change in Long-Term Care*, eds. Audrey S. Weiner and Judah Ronch (New York: Taylor and Francis, 2013), 53.

55 Benyamin Schwartz, *Nursing Home Design: Consequences for Employing the Medical Model* (New York: Garland Publishing, 1996).

56 Migette L. Kaup, Mark A. Proffitt, and Addie M. Abushousheh, "Building a 'Practice-Based' Research Agenda: Emerging Scholars Confront a Changing Landscape in Long-Term Care," *Journal of Housing for the Elderly* 26, no. 1–3 (2012): 94–120.

57 Robert A. Kane, "Long-Term Care and a Good Quality of Life: Bringing Them Closer Together," *The Gerontologist* 41, no. 3 (2001): 293–304.

58 Migette L. Kaup, "The Significance of the Door in Nursing Homes: A Symbol of Control in the Domestic Sphere," *Journal of Architectural Design and Domestic Space: Home Cultures* 8, no. 1 (2011): 25–42.

59 Migette L. Kaup and Gayle Doll, "Designing for Intimacy in Nursing Homes," *Implications* 10, no. 1 (2015), www.informedesign.org/Portals/0/Implications/Designing%20for%20Intimacy%20in%20Nursing%20Homes%20Vol%2010%20Issue%201.pdf.

60 Kaup, "The Significance of the Door in Nursing Homes."

61 Stephen L. Shields and Norton LaVrene, *In Pursuit of the Sunbeam: A Practical Guide to Transformation from Institution to Household* (Milwaukee, Wisconsin: Action Pact Press, 2006).

62 Anna N. Rahman and John F. Schnelle, "The Nursing Home Culture-Change Movement: Recent Past, Present, and Future Directions for Research (The Forum)," *The Gerontologist* 48, no. 2 (2008): 142–148.

63 Deborah Wilkerson and Christine MacDonell, "Quality Oversight and Culture Change in Long-Term Care," *Journal of Social Work in Long-Term Care* 2 (2003): 382.

64 Kaup and Doll, "Designing for Intimacy in Nursing Homes."

65 Kaup, Proffitt, and Abushousheh, "Building a 'Practice-Based' Research Agenda."

66 Sela Panapasa, James Jackson, Cleopatra Caldwell, Steve Heeringa, James McNally, David Williams, Debra Coral, Leafa Taumoepeau, Louisa Young, Setafano Young, and Saia

Fa'Asisila, "Community-Based Participatory Research Approach to Evidence-Based Research: Lessons From the Pacific Islander American Health Study," *Progress in Community Health Partnerships* 6, no. 1 (2012): 53–58.

67 "Accelerating HIV Treatment in the WHO Eastern Mediterranean and UNAIDS Middle East and North Africa Regions," World Health Organization Regional Office for the Easter Mediterranean, and UNAIDS, 2013, 24.

68 Benjamin Mason Meier and Ashley Fox, "International Obligations Through Collective Rights: Moving From Foreign Health Assistance to Global Health Governance," *Health and Human Rights* 12, no. 1 (2010): 61–72.

69 Laura Anderko, "Achieving Health Equity on a Global Scale Through a Community-Based, Public Health Framework for Action," *Journal of Law, Medicine & Ethics* 38, no. 3 (2010): 486–489.

70 "Accelerating HIV Treatment."

71 Panapasa et al., "Community-Based Participatory Research."

72 Mason Meier and Fox, "International Obligations Through Collective Rights."

73 "Accelerating HIV Treatment."

74 Mason Meier and Fox, "International Obligations Through Collective Rights."

75 Roger S. Ulrich, Robert F. Simons, Barbara D. Losito, Evelyn Fiorito, Mark A. Miles, and Michael Zelson, "A Conceptual Framework for the Domain of Evidence-Based Design," *Herd-Health Environments Research & Design Journal* 4, no. 1 (2010): 95–114.

16

THE INTERSECTION OF LAW, HUMAN HEALTH, AND BUILDINGS

Nicole DeNamur

Introduction

This chapter is organized into three sections: (1) brief historical background, (2) examples of regulatory issues involving buildings, and (3) discussion of themes and a precautionary approach. The historical background and examples are designed to prepare practitioners to identify issues and patterns, and plan for a changing future. The examples also highlight the role science plays in the legislative process, and demonstrate the need to shift away from a traditional, reactionary approach to regulation, and towards a proactive, precautionary approach.

Historical Background

Early in the history of regulation of buildings, threats to human health and safety, including massive fires and unsanitary living conditions, were relatively easy to pinpoint.[1] The regulatory responses were correspondingly narrow and reactionary. This reactionary approach is one of the reasons why the regulatory landscape, particularly in the United States, is so fragmented.[2]

Hammurabi's Code and the Bible

The following two examples illustrate that the design and construction of buildings has been governed by "rules" for a significant period of time.

King Hammurabi was a Babylonian ruler (1792–1750 B.C.) and author of the Code of Hammurabi.[3] Several sections of the Code are relevant to building design and construction, and generally outline a framework of responsibility through retaliation. For example, the Code provides that if the builder does not construct a house properly, and it falls and kills the owner, the builder will be killed.[4] If the house falls and kills the owner's son, the builder's son will be killed.[5] The Code also contains a section related to the builder's obligation to correct defective work. Paragraph 233 mandates that if the walls of a house appear to be toppling, even if the house is not complete, the builder must correct the work with his own labor and at his own expense.[6]

The King James Bible also contains rules that impact building design and safety. For example, among requirements related to various aspects of daily life is an apparent requirement that homes be constructed with a parapet on the roof.[7] A parapet, or barrier where the roof meets the walls of a structure, can prevent building occupants from falling from the roof.

London's Great Fire of 1666

In 1666, the Great Fire burned through London. Some sources estimate that one-third of the city was destroyed by the fire.[8] In response, the "1666 Act for rebuilding the City of London" attempted to mitigate the risk of future fires by mandating, among other things, that all houses be rebuilt with brick or stone (or a combination of the two), as opposed to flammable materials. The Great Fire literally reshaped the city, because these reactive requirements dictated how the structures that made up the city could be rebuilt. Other cities, including Seattle (1889) and Chicago (1871), responded to catastrophic fires by enacting similar building regulations.

High-Density Living Spaces in the Mid-1800s and Early 1900s

Numerous factors, including the Industrial Revolution, led to extremely dangerous and high-density living conditions on the East Coast of the United States in the mid-1800s.[9] According to some estimates, by 1900, as many as 2.3 million people (two-thirds of New York City's total population) lived in tenements.[10] Tenements are generally described as high-density, narrow, low-rise (five to seven stories) apartment buildings that take up nearly the entire lot.[11] At the time, building development was largely unregulated, and owners of tenement homes took advantage of the fact that they were not required to provide sanitary or even safe living conditions.[12] The severe overcrowding that tenements perpetuated posed numerous threats to human health, including a deadly cholera epidemic in New York City in 1849.[13]

To address this crisis, New York City enacted legislation governing tenement homes in the late 1800s and early 1900s. For example, The Tenement House Act of 1867 imposed requirements related to ventilation, fire escapes, banisters, toilets, cleaning, and reporting of infectious disease.[14] Subsequent, more robust legislation, including the Tenement House Act of 1901, contained additional requirements related to health and safety.[15]

Legislation governing tenement homes is one example of a shift in the regulatory framework to address not just life safety issues, but also the nexus between health and wellness, and the built environment. Courts supported these efforts by rejecting challenges to the validity of these new restrictions on private property owners. For example, in the early 1900s, a tenement house owner challenged the constitutionality of new regulations that required water closets, as opposed to unsanitary school sinks, in tenement homes. The Court emphasized the public health imperative in upholding the "preventative" regulations:

> We have here an act of the Legislature which is, in part, *preventative legislation, looking to the preservation of the public health in the future.* A system of drainage [a school sink] is attacked, which is highly dangerous, and which should be surrounded by every reasonable safeguard known to science and experts in plumbing.[16]

Examples of Regulatory Issues Related to Health, Safety, and Accessibility

Numerous economic, political, social, and other drivers shape the law. In turn, the law shapes the buildings where we live, work, and learn, and in light of the amount of time Americans spend indoors, the health and wellness of building occupants.

In the United States, regulation relevant to human health often centers on the question of what is "safe."[17] This question defies simple resolution and connects law, science, medicine, public policy, public health, and other related fields. The below examples demonstrate the issues and challenges faced by regulators, experts, and practitioners.

Drinking Water

In the United States, drinking water is highly regulated at the federal, state, and local levels. The existing paradigm is that, generally speaking, all water brought into a building, regardless of whether it will flow into a kitchen sink, bathtub, or toilet, must be "safe" to drink.[18] Certain water treatment and testing requirements originate from the Federal Safe Drinking Water Act of 1974 (SDWA).[19] The SDWA is a complicated piece of legislation that was significantly amended in 1986 and 1996, and applies to all public water systems.[20] Individual states, or other regulatory bodies, have authority to implement the many aspects of the SDWA within their borders.[21]

Under the SDWA, the Environmental Protection Agency (EPA) regulates drinking water by:

(1) identifying contaminants for potential regulation and determining which contaminants to regulate;
(2) setting a maximum contaminant level goal for each identified contaminant ("below which there is no known or expected risk to health"); and
(3) setting a maximum level for the contaminant or, if establishing a maximum is not economically or technically feasible, or no reliable or economic method to detect contaminants exists, setting a required treatment technique.[22]

The maximum level is an enforceable standard.[23]

Several sections of the SDWA highlight the connections between public health, science, and regulation, and demonstrate that what is considered "safe" can vary based on the circumstances and current body of scholarship:

Risk assessment, management, and communication

(A) Use of science in decisionmaking

In carrying out this section, and, to the degree that an Agency action is based on science, the Administrator shall use—

(i) the *best available, peer-reviewed science and supporting studies conducted in accordance with sound and objective scientific practices*; and

(ii) data collected by *accepted methods or best available methods* (if the reliability of the method and the nature of the decision justifies use of the data).[24]

This section is one example of how advancements in science can influence the regulatory framework, its interpretation, and enforcement.

To comply with certain aspects of the SDWA's mandates, and reduce the risks associated with waterborne illness, regulatory bodies often add chlorine to the water supply.[25] Historically, the positive impacts to human health as a result of regulation of drinking water—including chlorination—have been profound. In fact, in 1997, LIFE magazine featured the combination of filtration of drinking water and the use of chlorine in a special issue "The Millennium, 100 Events That Changed The World."[26] However, more recently, certain studies and groups have expressed concern regarding the potential negative health impacts of this process, and questioned whether this is still the most appropriate practice.[27] The question remains as to how the SDWA, and other regulations governing drinking water, may or may not evolve to address these, and other, concerns.

Toxic Building Materials: Lead and Asbestos

The following two examples demonstrate common building materials that negatively impact the health and wellness of building occupants.

Lead in Consumer Paints

Lead poisoning from exposure to or ingestion of lead-based paint, particularly in children, was the subject of significant public attention in the 1950s and 1960s and was widely considered to be a national public health issue.[28] It was not until 1978 that the federal government essentially banned the use of paint containing certain levels of lead for consumer uses.[29] The rationale for the ban provides insight regarding the regulatory control:

The [Consumer Product Safety] Commission has issued the ban because it has found that there is an *unreasonable risk* of lead poisoning in children associated with lead content of over 0.06 percent in paints and coatings to which children have access and that *no feasible consumer product safety standard under the CPSA would adequately protect the public from this risk.* The 0.06 percent is reduced to 0.009 percent effective August 14, 2009.[30]

However, these regulations fail to adequately protect families because they generally do not require remediation or abatement of homes with existing lead paint.[31] As a result, many children and families still suffer from impacts ranging from behavioral issues to permanent brain damage due to a *completely preventable disease.*[32] In fact, lead remains so pervasive in the built environment that federal law requires sellers and landlords to provide certain disclosures to purchasers and renters of homes built prior to 1978.

Lead is an interesting example for study because regulators somehow struggled to establish a level that was "safe" for a known toxin with the ability to cause both temporary and permanent harm to human health.[33] The dialogue regarding how to legally define "safe" was influenced by both industry groups, and the scientific and public health communities. As further discussed below, regulators will likely struggle with similar questions as the market demands increased transparency regarding the composition of many other common building products, some containing chemicals with known or suspected negative impacts to human health.

Asbestos

Asbestos is a naturally occurring mineral that has been used in a variety of building products ranging from insulation to floor tiles.[34] There are at least three primary health risks from inhaling high levels of asbestos fibers:

(1) lung cancer;
(2) mesothelioma; and
(3) asbestosis.[35]

There are two approaches to managing asbestos once it has been identified in the built environment: sealing or encapsulating the material so the fibers cannot escape, or completely removing the material (which could release fibers into the environment).[36]

During the 1970s, the EPA and Consumer Product Safety Commission banned various asbestos-containing products outright and in certain applications.[37] In July of 1989, the EPA exercised its rulemaking authority under the Toxic Substances Control Act (TSCA) and issued a broad-reaching final rule that banned the manufacture, importation, processing, and distribution of most products containing asbestos, and required labeling of these products.[38] In support of the original 1989 rule that was largely overturned, the EPA put forth the following supporting data: "The EPA estimates that this rule will save either 202 or 148 lives, depending upon whether the benefits are discounted, at a cost of approximately $450–800 million, depending upon the price of substitutes."[39] However, this rule was challenged by industry groups, and ultimately vacated in 1991 by the United States Court of Appeals for the Fifth Circuit.[40]

The practical result of industry pressure and the court's ruling was that only five products containing asbestos were ultimately banned (flooring felt, rollboard, and corrugated, commercial, or specialty paper),[41] and asbestos could not be used in products that did not historically contain the element ("new uses").[42] There are numerous other agencies and regulations that govern asbestos exposure, but contrary to popular belief, as of this writing, many products that contain asbestos can be legally manufactured and distributed in the United States, including clothing, cement shingles, and disk brake pads.[43] This could change as the Toxic Substances Control Act was revised in 2016, and, among other materials, asbestos regulation *could* be revised.[44]

Accessibility

While a comprehensive review of the Americans with Disabilities Act (ADA) is beyond the scope of this chapter, the ADA is a critical piece of civil rights legislation that must be a part of the conversation regarding regulation that impacts both buildings and human health and wellness. The ADA, related federal law, and associated implementing regulations shape buildings by improving accessibility to members of our communities.

The ADA was signed into law by President George H.W. Bush in the summer of 1990, and defines its purpose as:

(1) to provide a clear and comprehensive national mandate for the elimination of discrimination against individuals with disabilities;
(2) to provide clear, strong, consistent, enforceable standards addressing discrimination against individuals with disabilities;
(3) to ensure that the Federal Government plays a central role in enforcing the standards established in this chapter on behalf of individuals with disabilities; and
(4) to invoke the sweep of congressional authority, including the power to enforce the fourteenth amendment and to regulate commerce, in order to address the major areas of discrimination faced day-to-day by people with disabilities.[45]

The ADA covers many aspects of everyday life, and in order to carry out its directives, existing building codes and other regulations were impacted and new codes and regulations were enacted.[46]

The ADA does not specifically define who is entitled to protection, but instead defines "disability" as (1) a physical or mental impairment that substantially limits one or more major life activities; (2) a record of such an impairment; or (3) a person who is regarded by others as having such an impairment.[47] Major life activities include, among other things, performing manual tasks, standing, speaking, concentrating, and working.[48] Numerous regulations implement and provide detail for how the purpose and mandates of the ADA should be carried out from a practical standpoint, and various government entities are responsible for administration of these requirements.[49]

Themes and a Precautionary Approach

Analyzing Cyclical Themes

Law and science interact in important and dynamic ways. Science ultimately supports regulation, and as the collective knowledge base regarding the environmental and human health impacts of many common building materials continues to grow, these interactions will become more frequent. There are many regulatory challenges that complicate these issues, and practitioners may also question why, given the available data supporting the negative health impacts of lead and asbestos, regulation did not happen more quickly and comprehensively. In addition to legal complexities, industries with an interest in stalling regulation and discounting science played a role in lengthening the process.[50] Questioning of the science and scientists persists, as demonstrated by the many individuals and organizations that, despite the written scholarship, continue to deny the reality of climate change.[51]

The examples in this chapter represent cyclical themes and demonstrate the need for revisions to the regulatory framework to both drive change and support changing market and industry demands. For example, based largely on historical concerns related to both catastrophic fire and collapse, most jurisdictions place maximum height restrictions on various types of heavy timber construction. An increased awareness of the negative environmental impacts of construction materials that rose in popularity after the Industrial Revolution, including steel and concrete, led the industry to seek out alternative materials. This awareness also led to a discussion of whether existing height limitations are still appropriate for wooden structures, and consideration of relatively new forestry products such as cross-laminated timber (CLT).

Another example is the number of jurisdictions that have responded to an increasing demand for housing at urban centers by permitting "micro-housing" developments that support very high-density living. Among other issues, some communities have expressed concern that these high-density developments could foster the legal and social justice issues associated with tenement homes, mobile home parks, and public housing projects. Manufactured homes and mobile home parks, used to house an influx of temporary war workers, became increasingly prevalent in the United States during the 1940s.[52] Prefabricated structures, similar in many ways to mobile homes, are again being used, and in some cases stacked, to accommodate "micro-housing" development and construction in tight, urban spaces. These developments often house an influx of workers employed by industries experiencing rapid growth, such as technology companies. This cyclical pattern presents interesting questions and concerns regarding human health and wellness. For example, in high-density communities where some families are, for various reasons, unable or choosing not to vaccinate children, will certain diseases become more prevalent?

Finally, long-standing paradigms such as chlorination of drinking water, once seen as a remarkable public health advancement, are now being questioned in a different technological and public health climate. What will the future hold and what questions will future leaders struggle with as the intersection of law and public health continues to expand? There are, and will continue to be, many questions regarding how we define health and safety, including who decides, based on what science, and based on what volume of scientific evidence.[53] These questions will undoubtedly intersect with popular culture as new technology develops (and becomes less expensive) that allows us to monitor our health and environmental exposures with devices we can wear on our wrists or install in our homes.

Precautionary Regulation

Today, we are aware of, and exposed to, an increasing number of threats to our health and wellness. These threats range from exposure to toxins at relatively low, yet detrimental levels (or levels previously deemed "safe"), to the multi-faceted impacts of climate change. These threats require a different response, and a shift from reactionary, direct measures to proactive, sometimes indirect and precautionary measures to protect human health and wellness. They also require sophisticated science, strong economic support, motivated regulators and practitioners, and careful consideration of disproportionate impacts.

These considerations naturally lead to a discussion of the Precautionary Principle. An often-cited definition of the Precautionary Principle originates from the United Nations Conference on Environment and Development in June 1992, and the resulting Rio Declaration on Environment and Development. Principle 15 of the Declaration provides:

> In order to protect the environment, the precautionary approach shall be widely applied by States according to their capabilities. Where there are threats of serious or irreversible damage, lack of full scientific certainty shall not be used as a reason for postponing cost-effective measures to prevent environmental degradation.[54]

Unlike regulation in other parts of the world, regulation in the United States has generally operated contrary to the Precautionary Principle—presuming that chemicals or materials are safe until proven otherwise.[55] Making matters worse, there have been few requirements for testing prior to introduction into the consumer market, and when new regulations are passed, existing materials and chemicals are often grandfathered in, resulting in minimal, if any testing.[56] While this has historically been the case, there is some hope. As mentioned above, in 2016 the TSCA was revised in an effort to improve, among other things, the EPA's ability to regulate chemicals.[57]

Regulatory language that aligns with the Precautionary Principle is appropriate, particularly in light of the increasing volume of research and scholarship regarding the toxicity of materials and chemicals found in many common building products, fixtures, and furnishings, including formaldehyde, bisphenol A (BPA), and chemical flame-retardants.[58] As noted by the United States Court of Appeals for the District of Columbia Circuit, in analyzing the lead industry's challenge to federal efforts to regulate lead in gasoline pursuant to the Clean Air Act, "public health may properly be found endangered both by a lesser risk of a greater harm and by a greater risk of a lesser harm."[59] Industry groups and practitioners are driving change as they continue to demand increased transparency with regard to the composition of building products. Increased transparency is consistent with a precautionary approach, because, at a minimum, it supports more informed decision-making. We should continue to shift away from reactionary, direct measures and towards proactive, holistic, and sometimes indirect measures to protect human health and wellness, even though this shift will impact existing legislation and require leadership from government entities, corporations, and individuals.

Lessons learned from regulation of lead and asbestos can be extrapolated to other building components to improve the health and wellness of all individuals—from those working in the supply chain to building occupants—and reduce the risk to owners, designers, and builders of potential legal claims related to occupant health.[60] As part of this shift, careful attention must be paid to the disparate impacts of toxins on poor, marginalized, and minority populations.[61] Regulation must ensure that all individuals are provided with the *basic human right* of spaces to live, work, and learn that do not negatively impact human health. Practitioners should be guided by the principle that a building cannot be considered "healthy" if only certain groups have access to its benefits.

Finally, industry perspectives beyond law and public health need to be a part of this conversation and should be encouraged to take a leadership role. For example, financing and insurance institutions may be forced to consider changing frameworks for determining value and defining risk in light of the issues described in this chapter. These institutions will need to analyze how to value and insure conventional buildings against those that "improve," or at least do "less harm," to the health and wellness of their occupants through design. While these varied industries have not traditionally worked together, now is truly the time for collaboration. In fact, our health depends on it.

Disclaimer

This chapter is to be used for educational purposes only and is not intended to be, nor should it be construed as, legal advice or used as a legal reference. The laws, regulations, and policies described in this chapter are for illustrative and educational purposes only. As the law is constantly changing, this chapter is not intended to be, nor should it be used as, a source of information regarding the current state of the law. No warranty is made as to the completeness or accuracy of the information in this chapter.

Notes

1 Kevin Foy, "Home Is Where the Health Is: The Convergence of Environmental Justice, Affordable Housing, and Green Building," *Pace Environmental Law Review* (September 2012): 2.

2 A. P. Hurd and Al Hurd, *The Carbon Efficient City* (Seattle, WA: The University of Washington Press, 2012), 41–52; David Eisenberg and Sonja Persram, "Code, Regulatory and Systemic Barriers Affecting Living Building Projects," July 2009, 16, 27.

3 Centers for Disease Control and Prevention and U.S. Department of Housing and Urban Development, *Healthy Housing Reference Manual* (Atlanta: US Department of Health and Human Services, 2006), 3–1.

4 Leonard W. King, translator, *The Code of Hammurabi*, ¶ 229, by Hammurabi, King of Babylonia, contrib. by Charles F. Horne and C. H. W. Johns (http://avalon.law.yale.edu/ancient/hamframe.asp).

5 Ibid., ¶ 230.

6 Ibid., ¶ 233.

7 Deuteronomy 22:8, 21st Century King James.

8 Museum of London, "Infographic: The Great Fire of London," www.museumoflondon.org.uk/application/files/4714/5615/1274/fire-of-london-infographic.jpg.

9 CDC and U.S. Dept. of Housing, "Healthy Housing," 3–1.

10 History.com Staff, "Tenements," www.history.com/topics/tenements.

11 Ibid.

12 CDC and U.S. Department of Housing, "Healthy Housing," 3-1–3-2.

13 History.com Staff, "Tenements."

14 CDC and U.S. Department of Housing, "Healthy Housing," 3-1.

15 Ibid.

16 *Tenement House Department of the City of New York v. Moeschen*, 72 N.E. 231, 233–234 (1904), *aff'd per curiam*, 203 U.S. 583 (1906) (emphasis added).

17 Sarah Vogel, *Is It Safe? BPA and the Struggle to Define the Safety of Chemicals* (Los Angeles, CA: University of California Press, 2013).

18 Eisenberg and Persram, "Code, Regulatory and Systemic Barriers," 49.

19 Several sections of the SDWA, including those discussed in this chapter, and other sections related to lead, are (or may be) under review. For information and updates, consult the EPA's resources, including www.epa.gov/dwstandardsregulations/drinking-water-regulations-under-development-or-review.

20 United States Environmental Protection Agency, "Understanding the Safe Drinking Water Act," June 2004, www.epa.gov/sites/production/files/2015-04/documents/epa816f04030.pdf.

21 E.P.A., "Understanding the SDWA."

22 Ibid.

23 Ibid.

24 42 U.S.C. § 300g-1(b)(3) (emphasis added).

25 Joel Sisolak and Kate Spataro, "Toward Net Zero Water: Best Management Practices for Decentralized Sourcing and Treatment," March 2011, 13.

26 Neil Winokur, "The Millennium, 100 Events That Changed the World, No. 46 Water Purification," *LIFE Special Double Issue* (October 1997): 80.

27 Sisolak and Spataro, "Toward Net Zero," 13; International Living Future Institute™, Living Building Challenge 3.0™, 44.

28 Gerald Markowitz and David Rosner, *Lead Wars: The Politics of Sciences and the Fate of America's Children* (Los Angeles, CA: University of California Press, 2013), 5.

29 16 C.F.R. § 1303.1(a)(1)-(2), and (b).

30 16 C.F.R. § 1303.1(c) (emphasis added).

31 Markowitz and Rosner, *Lead Wars*, 119–121.

32 Ibid., 15, 44–45, 231.

33 Ibid., 12.
34 CDC and U.S. Dept. of Housing, "Healthy Housing," 5–13.
35 Ibid.
36 Ibid., 5–14.
37 United States Environmental Protection Agency, "U.S. Federal Bans on Asbestos," www2.epa.gov/asbestos/us-federal-bans-asbestos.
38 E.P.A., "Asbestos."
39 *Corrosion Proof Fittings v. E.P.A.*, 947 F.2d 1201, 1208 (5th Cir. 1991), *opinion clarified*, November 15, 1991.
40 E.P.A., "Asbestos;" *Corrosion Proof Fittings v. E.P.A.*, 947 F.2d at 1207.
41 40 C.F.R. § 763.165.
42 40 C.F.R. § 763.163 ("New uses of asbestos means commercial uses of asbestos not identified in §763.165 the manufacture, importation or processing of which would be initiated for the first time after August 25, 1989.")
43 E.P.A., "Asbestos."
44 *See* H.R. 2576, Public Law 114–182, Frank R. Lautenberg Chemical Safety for the 21st Century Act; U.S. Senate Environment and Public Works Committee, "Reforming the Toxic Substances Control Act."
45 42 U.S.C. § 12101(b).
46 Justin Sweet and Marc Schneier, *Legal Aspects of Architecture, Engineering and the Construction Process* (Stamford: Cengage Learning, 2013), 256–57.
47 42 USC § 12102 (1)(A)-(C).
48 42 USC § 12101 (2)(A).
49 Sweet and Schneier, *Legal Aspects*, 256; Barry Yatt, *Cracking the Codes: An Architect's Guide to Building Regulations* (New York: John Wiley & Sons), 41–43.
50 Markowitz and Rosner, *Lead Wars*, 226–228.
51 Ibid.
52 Allan Wallis, *Wheel Estate, the Rise and Decline of Mobile Homes* (Baltimore, M.D.: The Johns Hopkins University Press, 1997), 87–93.
53 Vogel, *Is It Safe*, 13–14; Markowitz and Rosner, *Lead Wars*, 219–223.
54 Text of the Rio Declaration, www.unep.org/Documents.multilingual/Default.asp?DocumentID=78&ArticleID=1163.
55 Vogel, *Is it Safe*, 6; Ian Urbania, "Think Those Chemicals Have Been Tested?" *The New York Times*, April 13, 2013, www.nytimes.com/2013/04/14/sunday-review/think-those-chemicals-have-been-tested.html; U.S. Senate Environment and Public Works Committee, "Reforming the Toxic Substances Control Act;" Puneet Kollipara, "The Bizarre Way the U.S. Regulates Chemicals—Letting Them on the Market First, Then Maybe Studying Them," *The Washington Post*, March 19, 2015, www.washingtonpost.com/news/energy-environment/wp/2015/03/19/our-broken-congresss-latest-effort-to-fix-our-broken-toxic-chemicals-law/.
56 Urbania, "Think Those Chemicals?"; Kollipara, "The Bizarre Way."
57 Kollipara, "The Bizarre Way;" U.S. Senate, "Reforming the TSCA;" H.R. 2576, Public Law 114–182, Frank R. Lautenberg Chemical Safety for the 21st Century Act.
58 Markowitz and Rosner, *Lead Wars*, 228–231.
59 *Ethyl Corp. et al. v. Environmental Protection Agency*, 541 F.2d 1, 18 (DC Cir. 1976).
60 Markowitz and Rosner, *Lead Wars*, 218–219.
61 Ibid., 230; Office of Healthy Homes and Lead Control, "Healthy Homes Survey, Lead and Arsenic Findings," ES-1–ES-2.

AFTERWORD

There is a truth stretching out across our design horizons which for some time many have suspected was true, a few have worked hard to understand, but most have quietly ignored. It offers enormous hope to the curious, threatens the paradigms of the comfortable, and motivates the willing to persevere. From many disciplines it invites a new blended intellectual realm between a crowded field of gifted design practitioners and researchers in nearly all sectors of human studies, scientific inquiry, and the natural and built environment. And it appears to be a truth so profound that it threatens to reshape not only the foundations of design practice, but potentially the very principles around which previously siloed curricula will soon find themselves fully integrated.

And That Truth???? Our Built and Natural Environments Influence Our Health and Well-being

What if the measure of our success as designers included the impact of our designs on human health? Dr. Richard Jackson, a noted health and well-being advocate, is fond of challenging audiences of design professionals as to whether or not they see themselves as health professionals. His point is simple: the places we designers create impact our health, so how can we best recognize and exploit this influence to the betterment of all?

Much has been said about the multidisciplinarity of this issue. Training and practice in design does not generally equip practitioners for the challenge of understanding the breadth of knowledge shared by all professions dedicated to health and well-being. For the design professional, a comfortable practice in or around this multi-dimensional field entails learning new languages, appreciating different approaches to research, tapping into extensive new libraries of research and reference materials in a host of new knowledge communities, all while maintaining practice and continuing education requirements for the original design competence.

The challenge of building a design practice with a multi-disciplinary world view is not a small one. While not a perfect indicator of the breadth of fields of knowledge, consider that CareerProfiles identifies 97 Associate and Bachelor undergraduate degrees. At the graduate level it lists 95 Master level degrees, and points out that in addition to four different kinds of Doctoral degrees there are also Professional and Specialist degrees.[1] Even after one acknowledges the potential relevance and impact of other knowledge disciplines on design, how does one know where or how to start to incorporate them into design thinking?

Even a cursory scan of the Table of Contents for this text shows very quickly the number of different disciplines being brought to bear on the subject of designing interiors for health and well-being. It is inconceivable that any design professional could amass command of a sufficient number of the knowledge areas to be considered an expert in all. And this brings me to my first main point:

> Multidisciplinarity is not the point; the thoughtful and careful integration of multiple disciplines into singular solutions is the point.

Multi-disciplinary environments surround us all. For example, our kitchens represent a multi-disciplinary blank canvas. We have refrigerated goods, dry goods, spices, oils, a variety of containers, assorted cooking tools, frozen goods, and several different kinds of appliances for cooking and cleaning up after our creations. And don't forget the inventory of serving dishes, plates, cups, silverware, and condiments that rightly accompany the dining experience. Being surrounded by so many different food-related components is not what matters; rather, it is the magic of integrating them in a recipe of proportions and sequencing, providing the proper preparation, and plating the results for optimal visual pleasure that creates the wonder of a culinary delight. And let's be honest—can't you recall a time when you had a multi-disciplinary dish that you vowed to never have again?

> Integration, alone, is not the point. Integration is a means within a multi-disciplinary world, and when it is done right, it is magical.

Don't think that the migration to integrative thinking is a fad, unworthy of serious consideration. Siloed knowledge is no longer perceived with the same value proposition as in years past. Many research frontiers are driven by the premise that integrated multi-disciplinary solutions are the only way to deal with multi-faceted complex issues. One can even pursue formal study in the art and science of integration. BestColleges.Com identifies 37 colleges and universities that offer majors and study curricula for individuals who want to build careers in the integration of multiple knowledge sets.[2] Integration is an art, and science, unto itself.

And here is the good news: design professionals are perhaps the most naturally gifted integrators on the planet, and fortunately the academic and practical training they experience during their careers only further this natural gift. It is, quite simply, what they do. Design professionals routinely integrate knowledge bases on materials, budgets, building codes, fire codes, environmental constraints, engineering recommendations, construction methods and materials, accessibility guidelines, and a myriad of other design influences. It is a perfectly natural and thoroughly manageable step to welcome health and well-being into the design experience and embrace its potential to raise design to new performance levels for occupants. This brings me to my second main point:

> Designing for health and well-being requires that we adjust our traditional design thinking.

The first adjustment to which I will point is a distinction that is becoming more prominent in the design conversation: designing to avoid toxicity or risk to human health is not the same as designing for enhanced health. For example, one avoids toxicity when the building materials that off-gas formaldehyde or other potentially hazardous volatile organics are avoided in the construction process, or when the risk of asbestos exposure is managed by its removal or other remediation techniques. The design objective is to do no harm, and is instead, by removing or controlling the environmental hazards, to create a neutral environment that doesn't endanger the health of occupants. Today, we understand that this approach does not go far enough in the matter of designing for a positive impact on human health and well-being.

Design that enhances the health and well-being of occupants is salutogenic design, a term derived from the work of Dr. Aaron Antonovsky in which he coined the term "salutogenesis."[3] In this case the design objective is to create environments that actually improve the physical, intellectual, emotional, and spiritual health of occupants. Research done by Dr. Roger Ulrich in the early 1980s demonstrated how a view from a hospital room could improve the physical health of patients such that they needed less pain medications and had shorter lengths of stay as recovering inpatients.[4] Research currently being done at Harvard by Dr. Joseph Allen and others shows that increased air ventilation rates actually improve mental function.[5] This is design that goes beyond simply being non-toxic; it is health-enhancing. It is a design frontier that demands our full attention.

The second adjustment to our design thinking that I will propose is that we must find a way to add health and well-being outcome metrics to our projects. Since 1948 the World Health Organization has suggested that a definition of health must reach beyond simply not being sick,[6] but what are the metrics to define and monitor health and well-being? How do we scale and measure outcomes like satisfaction, contentment, or quality of life? How will we know if our designs have succeeded in having the intended beneficial impact to health and well-being? To do this we must make certain that we know which health and well-being outcomes we want to impact, how we will measure that impact, and importantly for the design community, how we propose to impact them with design.

Designing for a health or well-being outcome is in some ways little differ-ent than designing for an energy utilization profile; the various factors impacting energy use are identified, studied, and incorporated into the design with a perfor-mance expectation derived perhaps from modeling and/or relevant research. The same might be said of designing for a desired acoustic experience by a building occupant; doing the requisite study of building materials, sound attenuation factors, and intended building uses, and then incorporating those findings into the design process to produce a solution that achieves the desired acoustic performance result. We must make the same effort in health and well-being outcomes, serving, again, as master integrators of those knowledge pools with design. The contributors to this book are openly suggesting that the knowledge integration that they have pursued linking health and well-being outcomes and design processes can favorably impact design and its beneficial impact on building users. That is a powerful premise of inestimable potential value.

Another adjustment that I will propose to our design thinking is that we must refine our evaluation of design for health and well-being to accommodate the vagaries of those particular outcome metrics. For example, anyone who has pursued improved health in a gym or on a track knows that improvements sometimes come slowly, over time, and often with extended effort and little visible result. Such can be the case with design for enhanced health and well-being, where sometimes the results are slow to arrive. And a design that is conscientiously non-toxic might be highly successful in not making people sick, but how challenging is it to measure success of design by the non-occurrence of illness? Conversely, how immediately obvious is it that an environment is toxic when an occupant reacts to an allergen or toxin with a violent, acute response to that stimulus? It is important that any post-occupancy evaluation of the success of a deliberate attempt to design for health and well-being be sensitive to the variation among possible outcomes.

Lastly, we must adjust our design thinking to be mindful of the price we are paying for our healthy designs and not allow our pursuit of the possible to blindly overpower the pursuit of the practical. While it is important to prioritize our health and well-being, it is likewise important to balance those costs against a host of other design parameters, including, for example, effective functionality, pleasing form and aesthetic, and a reasonable understanding of the timeframe for realizing the benefit imagined during the design experience.

Just following developments in this field requires an appreciation for emerging multi-disciplinary linkages and the requisite integrative skills needed to achieve their full value. Participating in this design wave demands revisiting familiar design models, and refusing to do things just "because they've always been done that way." In this book writers from a great variety of backgrounds have contributed to the multi-disciplinary discourse around the ways that the built and natural environ-ments impact our health and well-being. I encourage you to read on and lend your voice to the conversation as an integrator, as an innovator, and as an instigator of change in this important field that intimately touches and impacts every one of us.

A. Ray Pentecost III

Notes

1 "Types of College Degrees," CareerProfiles, Career and Job Search Guide, www.career profiles.info/types-of-college-degrees.html.

2 "Best Integrative Studies Programs," BestColleges.com, www.bestcolleges.com/features/top-integrative-studies-programs/.

3 Aaron Antonovsky, *Unraveling the Mystery of Health: How People Manage Stress and Stay Well* (San Francisco, CA: Jossey-Bass Social and Behavioral Science Series and The Jossey-Bass Health Series,1987): 218.

4 Roger S. Ulrich, "View Through a Window May Influence Recovery From Surgery," *Science* 224, no. 4647 (April 27, 1984): 420–1.

5 Piers MacNaughton, James Pegues, Usha Satish, Suresh Santanam, John Spengler, and Joseph Allen, "Economic, Environmental and Health Implications of Enhanced Ventilation in Office Buildings," *International Journal of Environmental Research and Public Health* 12 (2015): 14709–22.

6 Preamble to the Constitution of the World Health Organization as adopted by the *International Health Conference*, New York, 19–22 June 1946; signed on 22 July 1946 by the representatives of 61 States (Official Records of th World Health Organization, no. 2, p. 100) and entered into force on 7 April 1948.

INDEX